DAMN FINE
CHERRY PIE

THE UNAUTHORIZED COOKBOOK
INSPIRED BY THE TV SHOW *TWIN PEAKS*

DAMN FINE CHERRY PIE

THE UNAUTHORIZED COOKBOOK
INSPIRED BY THE TV SHOW *TWIN PEAKS*

by Lindsey Bowden

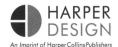

HARPER DESIGN
An Imprint of HarperCollinsPublishers

This publication has not been prepared, approved or
licensed by any entity or individual that created or produced
the well-known TV program *Twin Peaks*.

First published in Great Britain in 2016 by Mitchell Beazley, an imprint of Octopus Publishing Group Ltd,
Carmelite House, 50 Victoria Embankment, London EC4Y 0DZ www.octopusbooks.co.uk

DAMN FINE CHERRY PIE

Published in 2016 by
Harper Design
An Imprint of HarperCollinsPublishers
195 Broadway
New York, NY 10007
Tel: (212) 207-7000
Fax: (855) 746-6023
harperdesign@harpercollins.com
www.hc.com

Distributed throughout North America by
HarperCollins *Publishers*
195 Broadway
New York, NY 10007

ISBN 978-0-06-249555-6

Library of Congress Control Number: 2016946279

Printed in China

First Printing, 2016

Commissioning Editor: Eleanor Maxfield; Art Director: Yasia Williams-Leedham; Senior Editor: Leanne Bryan;
Photographer: Addie Chinn; Food and Props Stylist: Annie Nichols; Designer: John Round; Copy Editor: Joanna Smith;
Picture Research Manager: Giulia Hetherington; Picture Library Manager: Jen Veall; Production Manager: Caroline Alberti

The 3 of Hearts on page 194, Louise Holland, courtesy of The Double R Club.

This book is dedicated to my wonderful Mum and Dad

Dad – your hard work and commitment to your family has inspired me
to be the best that I can be. I love you.

Mum – who I miss very much, who supported, encouraged, and believed
in me constantly, and who couldn't cook a damn thing! I love you.

CONTENTS

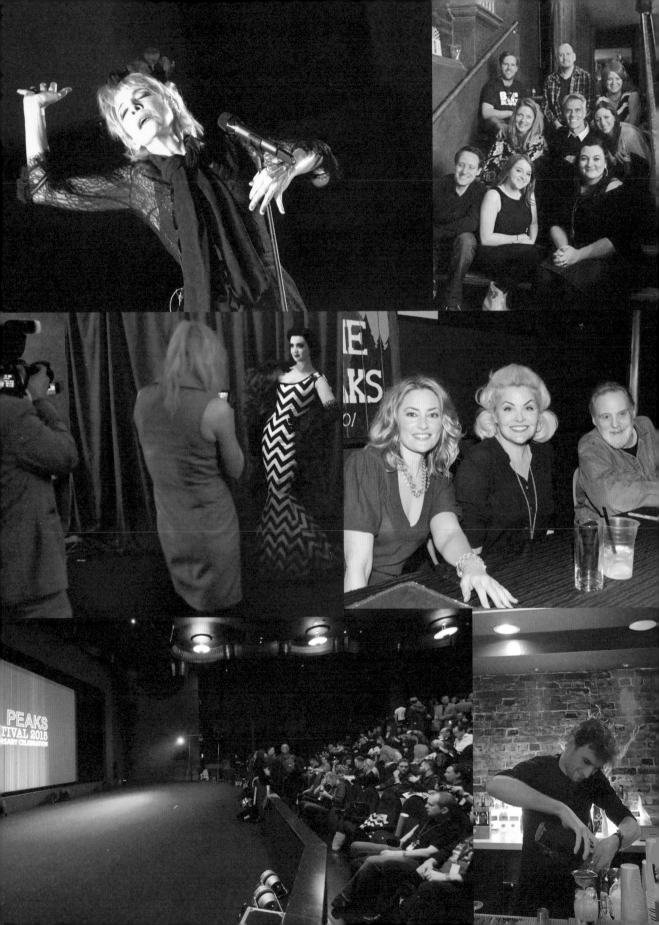

INTRODUCTION

It was 1990 and I was 14 years old when *Twin Peaks* first aired in the UK. I was addicted from the start. From the blinking BBC2 logo which led into the haunting theme tune, I was hooked. I was fascinated by this small town where nothing was as it seemed and everyone was asking the same question: Who killed Laura Palmer?

Fastforward to 2009 and, at the age of 33, working as a Producer in the film and theatre industry, I was still obsessed with the show. I had fallen so deeply in love with this fictitious world, I felt like I knew every corner of it.

One day, while working from home with an episode of *Twin Peaks* flickering away in the background, it struck me that the following year was the 20th anniversary of my favourite series. Yet there were no celebrations taking place in the UK. Why would there be? Was a 20-year-old show at the forefront of anyone's mind? But I knew the impact *Twin Peaks* had had on me, and how many fans were still out there. I decided to do something, for all of us, and created the *Twin Peaks* UK Festival. The idea was simple: include guests from the show, screenings and performances, and engulf fans in the world of *Twin Peaks* and David Lynch.

From that first event in 2010, the festival has grown. We have just celebrated our 6th annual festival with a special event dedicated to the 25th anniversary of *Twin Peaks*. And the festival continues to grow.

Food plays a crucial role in the *Twin Peaks* universe and I am always inspired to grab a bite to eat when watching the programme. I love cooking and the idea of food as an experience, from styling and setting to texture and flavours – it should be a celebration. I wanted to bring my interpretation of the food in *Twin Peaks* to life in the real world and so I began to write this cookbook – a perfect way to unite my two passions.

In this book you will find all your *Twin Peaks* favourites, as well as recipes that have been inspired by characters, storylines and locations. There are food symbols that are important to the programme: the cherry pie served at the RR Diner, the donuts in the Sheriff's Department and the Great Northern breakfasts – not to mention coffee. No cookbook would be complete without these favourites, but there is so much more to explore.

I wanted to play around with the idea of food that is wholesome and American on the surface – tempting, comforting and classic – but also explore the darker, more seductive themes in the programme. Using the locations and characters as a foundation, I started to devise recipes such as hearty breakfasts and a diner menu that would celebrate 1950s American culture. I got carried away with an extensive list of pastries and donuts to whet your appetite and share with friends. I thought about how fans love to immerse themselves in the world of *Twin Peaks*, and the recent trend for hosting supper clubs and themed dinner parties. I created a White Lodge chapter that summarized a sense of safety, purity and family life. And I created a Black Lodge dinner chapter full of richer, darker, moodier recipes to set the scene. Finally there are a host of cocktails to get your party started with a swing – the perfect way to toast your favourite show.

The *Twin Peaks* UK Festival continues to grow and grow. Over the years we have been joined by some incredible guests from the show, including Sheryl Lee, Dana Ashbrook, Madchen Amick,

Sherilyn Fenn, Catherine E. Coulson, Al Strobel, Charlotte Stewart, Lenny Von Dohlen, Phoebe Augustine, Kimmy Robertson, Ian Buchanan and Julee Cruise, who has performed live twice at the festival.

As those of you who have been to the *Twin Peaks* UK Festival know, we relish the idea of surrounding you in the world of *Twin Peaks*. My intention is to do the same with these recipes – bringing that wonderful world into your own home to share with friends.

I am honoured to have the opportunity to combine two of my great passions, *Twin Peaks* and food, and to bring you this little slice of *Twin Peaks*-inspired culinary heaven. I sincerely hope you have as much fun cooking these recipes as I did creating them!

Hang loose Haoles!

The fictional town of Twin Peaks is actually the towns of North Bend, Snoqualmie and Fall City in Washington State. Just down the road is Roslyn, the town where *Northern Exposure* was filmed.

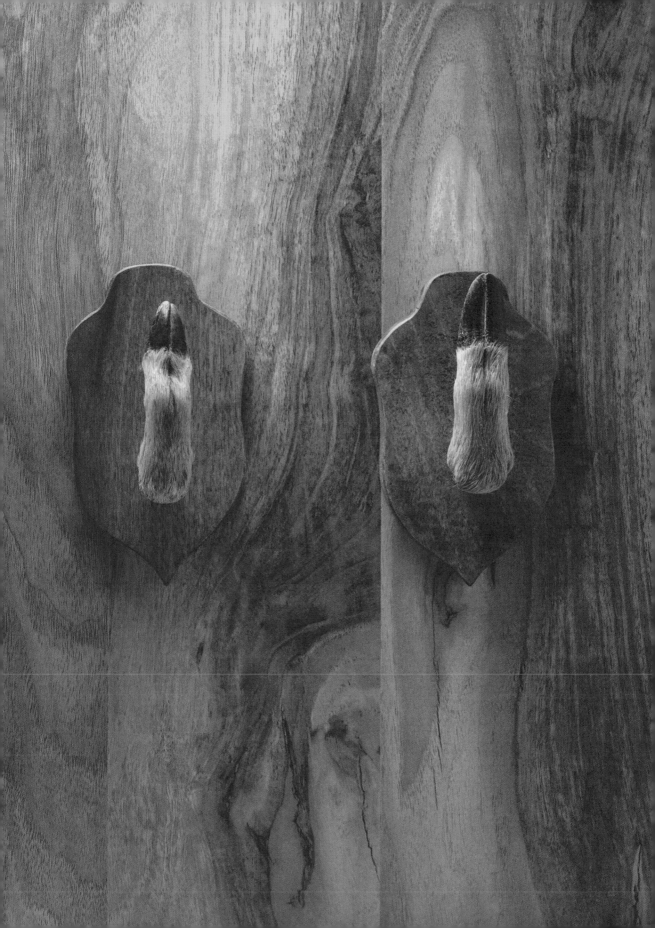

"THE BEST TV SHOW EVER MADE"

24 February 1989 and the lifeless body of Laura Palmer, wrapped in plastic, washes up next to a giant log, in the town of Twin Peaks.

This simple idea from co-creators David Lynch and Mark Frost created a television show that turned into a cult phenomenon. A brutal murder, a small American town and nothing is quite as it seems.

David Lynch was known as a film director who created surreal, almost nightmarish movies such as *Eraserhead* and *Blue Velvet*. Mark Frost was a television writer known mostly for his sterling work on *Hill Street Blues*. With the unique mix of Lynch's abstractism and Frost's insight into everyday America, it seemed the perfect match to create this town and indeed this world.

Twin Peaks first aired on April 8 1990 in the USA and six months later in the UK. It ran for two seasons before being cancelled by ABC due to declining figures, figures which only declined after Lynch was asked by the network to reveal who the killer was part-way through Season 2.

However, even though the series had been cancelled, a prequel movie followed, *Twin Peaks: Fire Walk With Me* with Robert Engels on board as co-writer and David Lynch back at the helm as director as well as co-writer.

Initially panned by the critics, *FWWM* (as Peakies lovingly refer to it) has become something of a cult classic and is considered by many to be the masterpiece of Lynch's films.

And 25 years later, we're still talking about it, we're still theorizing over it, and the show itself is making a welcome return to our screens in 2017. At the time of writing, the new *Twin Peaks* (or is it Season 3…) is currently in production. The recipes contained in this book are inspired by the TV show, but it has not been prepared, approved or licensed by any entity or individual that created or produced the show.

So what is it that makes *Twin Peaks* so special? Is it the innovative writing? Is it the dynamic combination of a cast of young professionals such as Sheryl Lee, Sherilyn Fenn and Madchen Amick with older veterans of the acting world such as Piper Laurie, Russ Tamblyn and Richard Beymer? Or is it simply because it allows us to enter a world we'd never seen before? *Twin Peaks* has pushed boundaries and inspired writers from the time of airing right up until the present day.

TWIN PEAKS *AWARDS*

1990 Emmy Awards

- Outstanding Achievement in Costuming for a Series – Patricia Norris
- Outstanding Editing for a Series – Duwayne Dunham

1990 Grammy Awards

- Best Pop Instrumental Performance – Angelo Badalamenti, *Twin Peaks Theme Tune*

1990 Television Critics Association Awards

- Program of the Year
- Outstanding Achievement in Drama

2015 Saturn Awards

- Best DVD/BD Television Release – *Twin Peaks: The Entire Mystery*

1990 Casting Society of America Artios Awards

- Dramatic Episodic Casting – Johanna Ray

1991 Golden Globe Awards

- Best Drama TV Series
- Best Actor in a Drama TV Series – Kyle MacLachlan
- Best Supporting Actress in a Series – Piper Laurie

FACTS ABOUT TWIN PEAKS

1 *Twin Peaks* is often referred to as "The best TV show ever made!"

Twin Peaks *was originally going to be called Northwest Passage.* 2

3 The late Frank Silva, who plays BOB, was cast in the role after his reflection was accidentally caught in a mirror on camera. He was actually the set carpenter.

The late Jack Nance, who played Pete Martell, was in David Lynch's first feature film 4 *Eraserhead*, as was Charlotte Stewart who played Betty Briggs in *Twin Peaks*. Jack Nance was married to Log Lady Catherine E. Coulson at the time.

5 *David Lynch and Mark Frost also created the sitcom* On The Air *together, starring Ian Buchanan in the lead role before he took the role of Dick Tremayne in* Twin Peaks.

The fictional town of Twin Peaks is actually the towns of North Bend, Snoqualmie and 6 Fall City in Washington State. Just down the road is Roslyn, the town where *Northern Exposure* was filmed.

7 The book that accompanied the television show, *The Secret Diary of Laura Palmer*, was written by David Lynch's daughter, director Jennifer Lynch, when she was only 22 years old.

David Lynch did not want to reveal the killer of Laura Palmer but was asked to do so 8 *by the network. Ratings declined during Season 2, and* Twin Peaks *was cancelled after only two seasons.*

9 Richard Beymer (Ben Horne) and Russ Tamblyn (Dr Jacoby) also starred together in the 1961 film version of *West Side Story* as Tony and Riff.

The Log Lady was an idea formed in David Lynch's mind long before *Twin Peaks*. As far back as 10 *Eraserhead*, he and Catherine E. Coulson were discussing the character.

11 *The character of Madeleine Ferguson comes from Missoula, Montana, which is David Lynch's hometown.*

The house used for exterior shots of Laura Palmer's home changed between the pilot episode 12 and the prequel film *Twin Peaks: Fire Walk With Me*. The house used in the pilot was in the town of Monroe, north of Fall City, but the one used in the film was in Everett, north of Seattle. The interior of the Everett house was used as the Palmer house in both.

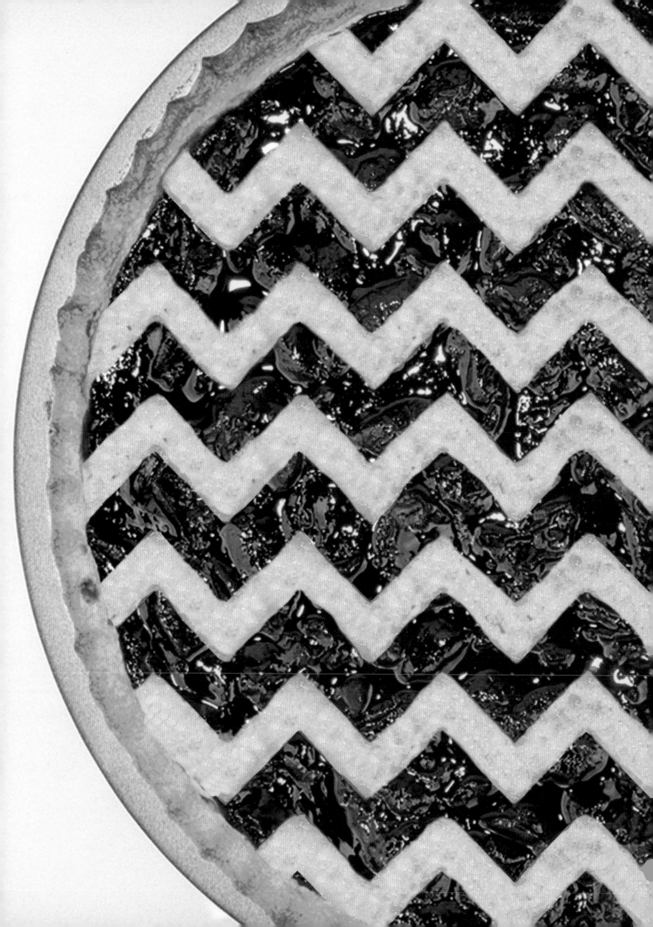

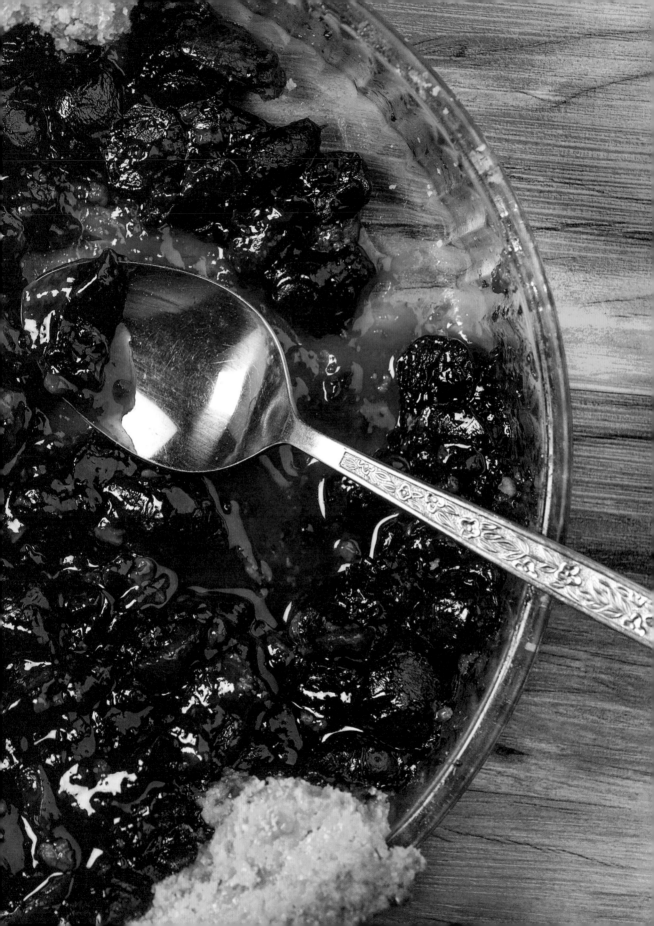

13 Kyle MacLachlan doesn't like cherry pie, so during the filming of *Twin Peaks* he is eating berry pie.

14 *James Marshall, who portrayed the character of James Hurley, really does play the guitar and really did sing the song "Just You" in* Twin Peaks.

15 The chevron floor of the Black Lodge in *Twin Peaks* also appears in Lynch's first feature film *Eraserhead*. It is the lobby floor of Henry's house.

16 The chess game corpse in the Sheriff's station was played by Kyle Maclachlan's brother Craig.

17 *Hank Jennings' prison number was the same as that of Jean Valjean from* Les Miserables *– 24601.*

18 The character of Josie Packard was originally going to be Italian and rumoured to be played by Isabella Rossellini.

19 *Twin Peaks* co-creator Mark Frost has a cameo in *Twin Peaks* playing a news reporter after the Packard sawmill fire.

20 *As well as playing husband and wife in* Twin Peaks, *Everett McGill and Wendy Robie (Ed and Nadine Hurley) teamed up again in the 1992 Wes Craven horror film,* The People Under the Stairs.

21 Zooey Deschanel's mother Mary Jo played Eileen Hayward in *Twin Peaks* and her father Caleb was a director on the show.

22 The station wagon that Al Strobel (AKA Mike) drives in *Fire Walk With Me* is actually his own vehicle. He thought his vehicle suited the film a lot better than the original car that was to be used. He still drives the same station wagon to this day.

23 *The strange way the characters talk in the Black Lodge was achieved by getting the actors to speak their lines backwards, then reversing the sound so they were being said the correct way.*

24 Warren Frost who plays Will "Doc" Hayward is actually the father of *Twin Peaks* co-creator Mark Frost.

25 Sheryl Lee, who plays Laura, was the original choice for the role of Mary Alice Young in *Desperate Housewives*. That role eventually went to Brenda Strong who also starred in *Twin Peaks* as the woman who tried to kill Sheriff Truman.

HOW TO THROW A DINNER PARTY INSPIRED BY TWIN PEAKS

Three words leap into my mind when I think of the world of *Twin Peaks* – detail, detail, detail! It's so important when something is as unique as *Twin Peaks* to really immerse people into that unique realm and transport them into another dimension. It's something you can put into practice at your own *Twin Peaks*-inspired dinner party.

First you need to choose a theme. Is it generic *Twin Peaks* or is it a Black Lodge special? Here are some suggestions:

- The Black Lodge residents
- The Sheriff's department
- A *Fire Walk With Me* special
- *Twin Peaks* High School
- *Twin Peaks* local businesses
- One Eyed Jacks
- A White Lodge interpretation

For the purposes of this book, we're going to look at a dinner party inspired by *Twin Peaks*. It goes without saying that your dinner party must have characters and therefore your guests must dress up. Whether they decide to be a character or an object, it's imperative that they look the part. If your guests don't know *Twin Peaks*, either uninvite them immediately, or give them a few helpful pointers: blue roses, cherries, log brooches...

DECOR

Wherever you choose to have your dinner party, the decor is the key element. This can be done pretty simply. A *Twin Peaks* staple has to be red drapes, so start the experience by having red drapes in the dining room. Your drapes don't have to be full-on velour theatre drapes, you can of course visit a fabric shop or even better a local market (if they have fabric stalls) and grab yourself some great red fabric at a really reasonable price. And of course a lighter fabric will be a lot easier to hang! The next essential is to make yourself a great "Welcome to *Twin Peaks*" sign to hang outside the front door.

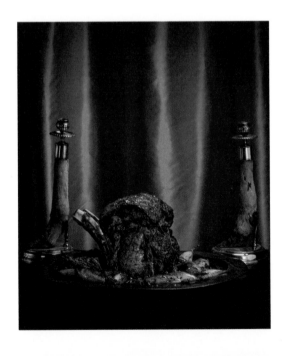

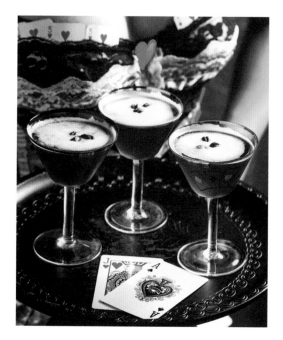

– owls, stag heads, and if you really want to go to town maybe a white fox or two! And of course no dinner party is complete without the guest of honour – so make sure you have a framed Laura Palmer homecoming queen photo in pride of place.

Another big theme in *Twin Peaks* is wood. Look at all the wood references – log trucks, the woods themselves, the diner walls – it's everywhere. A really simple way to bring this into your dinner party is to use wooden place mats and coasters – alongside your chevron table runner and red drapes you're already creating your own *Twin Peaks* set!

As much as I would love to tell you all to immediately convert your beautiful wooden floors or carpets to a gleaming black and white chevron floor, this is rather impractical. So a great way to keep the Black Lodge look is work the chevrons into everyday items. This is where Ebay is your best friend. There is a huge amount of chevron party wear on Ebay, including straws, paper plates, cups, napkins, table runners and even candles. You can also find chevron fabric on Ebay so if you feel like being extra fancy there is the option of covering your dining chairs too!

Extra accessories add to the authenticity of the experience, so go through your *Twin Peaks* box sets and pick out background items that really say "Peaks" to add to your decor. Some examples of these are the animals of *Twin Peaks*

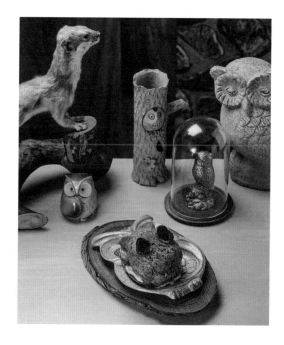

ENTERTAINMENT

As your guests arrive it's important that there's always music in the air so whack on your *Twin Peaks* soundtrack and the stage is set. Be ready to greet your guests with a nice cocktail – maybe the Audrey Horne's American Belle in the last chapter of this book – just to sweeten things up ready for the evening.

Entertainment is, of course, very important for any dinner party and, providing the weather is warm enough, you can't get any better than Tibetan Rock Throwing. A word of warning: don't use real glass or sugar glass! The clearing up and health and safety aspect will dampen the spirit. Plastic bottles will work just fine but try to collect a variation of sizes and stick to clear, brown and green bottles. Pour some water into the bottles so they don't blow over in the wind.

You needn't spend a fortune trying to find logs for your Tibetan Rock Throwing set, and it's probably best not to steal them from a public park. However, if you have woods near your home, contact the owner and ask to borrow a few logs to really create the atmosphere you need. They will probably be happy for you to take them off their hands. Of course you could go one step further and take the rock throwing to the woods – that's your choice!

For extra fun, you can add some prizes to your rock throwing and even learn Agent Cooper's opening Tibetan speech – as Benjamin Louche of The Double R Club (*see* pages 212–13) performs at the *Twin Peaks* UK Festival – if you want to really set the mood. Just don't forget the coffee and donuts.

Some other ideas for entertainment are:

*   *Twin Peaks* karaoke
*   *Twin Peaks*/David Lynch quiz (you are, of course, the quizmaster)
*   Soap in a sock throwing contest (possibly best for the garden)
*   Origami owl folding contest (*see* page 42 for instructions)

When it comes to food, there is an abundance of delicious dishes in this book, but be sure to finish feeding your guests on a damn fine cup of Good Morning America (in the evening…) and a selection of donuts. Then clear the dance floor and end the night with your favourite *Twin Peaks* character dance… Audrey Horne in the diner, Ben Horne tapping on his desk or Leland Palmer well, doing anything anywhere – it's all damn fine!

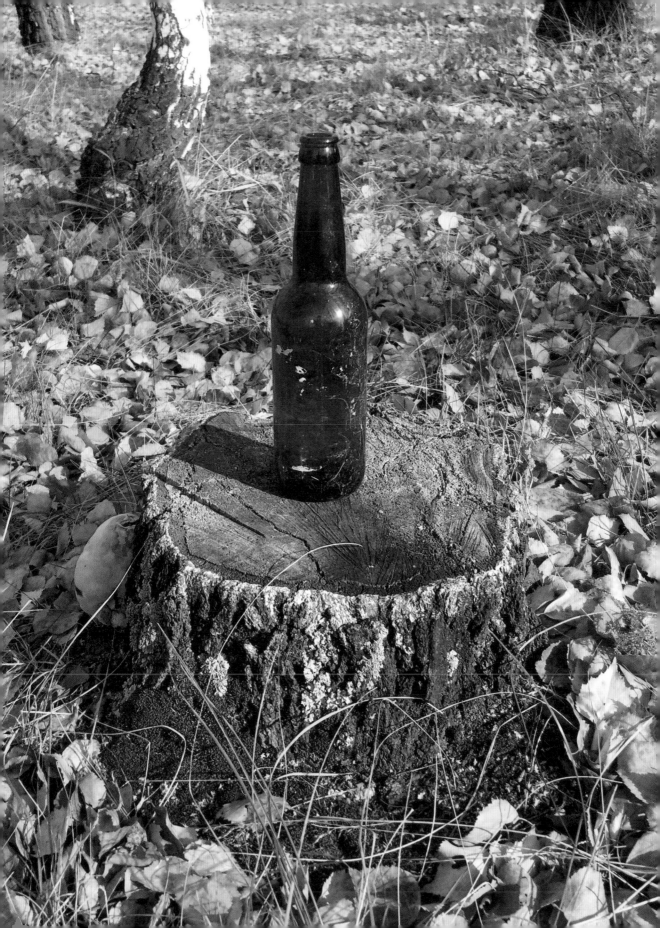

FASHION INSPIRED BY TWIN PEAKS

One thing that stands out about *Twin Peaks* is its timelessness. We all know the original series aired in 1990, but watch it today and not much dates it back to that time. Part of its timelessness is due to the costume design, masterminded in the pilot by the late Patricia Norris.

We have put together a little guide on how to achieve your favourite character's look. Whether it's the sultry siren allure of Audrey Horne or the girl-next-door style of Donna Hayward, we've got something for every Peakie!

AUDREY HORNE

That hair, those eyes, that smile… is there anything not to adore about *Twin Peaks* femme fatale, Audrey Horne? Mixing schoolgirl fashion with forties diva, Audrey, portrayed brilliantly by Sherilyn Fenn, combines seductiveness with femininity, creating possibly the most copied of the female *Twin Peaks* styles.

When we first meet Audrey Horne she is wearing a classic Audrey outfit: checked three-quarter-length skirt, pale pink sweater and black and white brogue-style pumps…which she quickly swaps for a pair of striking red heels out of her locker. Throughout the first season, Audrey wears a variation on this outfit but in Season 2, after her stint in One Eyed Jacks, Audrey starts to help with the family business and we see her fashion start to mature. In come the business suits and heels and the instantly recognizable coiffed hairdo. We have picked out a few staple items to help you achieve the cherished look of Ms Horne.

- Pleated checked three-quarter-length skirt
- Straight black three-quarter-length pencil skirt

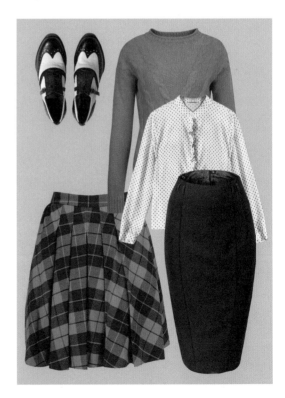

- Button-up, waist-length grey cardigan (with black trees on if you can find it!)
- Coloured, fitted, waist-length sweater with lace panelling across the collar, neck and upper chest
- Pale pink waist-length sweater
- Deep red sweater with loose, turtle-neck collar
- Sky blue, ribbed turtle-neck sweater
- Classic black tailored skirt suit (with skirt just above the knee)
- Black and white dogtooth coat with large collar
- Black and white brogue-style pumps
- Classic red heels
- Classic black court shoes with medium heel

And remember to plug in those heated curlers to achieve Audrey's famous hairstyle!

DONNA HAYWARD

Her best friend is leading a double life of the highest order, so it stands to reason that Donna Hayward is the juxtaposition to Laura and is a typical girl next door with a fashion sense to match. We're not saying Donna doesn't know how to turn it up – especially while trying to seduce James Hurley through those jail bars – but Donna tends to lean towards comfort and warmth. Try these items to achieve your Donna look – just remember not to borrow anything of Lauras!

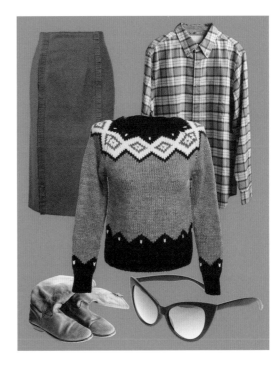

- Above-the-knee straight black skirt
- Oversized, grey three-quarter-length denim skirt
- Straight-leg dark-wash denim jeans
- Oversized grey cardigan with shape pattern (preferably diamonds)
- Bright orange chunky sweater
- Checked fitted shirt with collar
- Dark green checked waistcoat
- Cream fitted waist-length sweater with cream and brown striped scarf
- Brown suede jacket with collar (if you can find one with tassels on the front, even better!)
- Cream shirt with pixie collar and black embroidered flowers
- Flat brown leather ankle boots
- Flat black lace-up pumps

SHELLY JOHNSON

She dropped out of high school and married misogynist Leo Johnson, but Shelly is still one of the most desirable women in the town of Twin Peaks. Of course she is rarely seen out of her RR Diner uniform but when she is, she displays the look of an unhappy woman, scared in her home but secretly sharing her affection elsewhere. Throughout Season 2, after Leo breaks out of his coma and runs off into the woods, Shelly begins to use her feminine charms more and this shows through her attire.

To Shelly-up your wardrobe, try the following items:

- Grey crew-neck T-shirt
- Black waist-length button-up cardigan (mainly worn undone over a T-shirt)

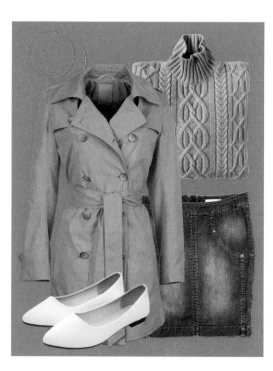

- Dark checked bath robe
- Sheer white chiffon shirt with a pattern up the front
- Black, long-sleeved, three-quarter-length jersey dress
- Grey cable knitted jumper
- Straight stonewash denim skirt – sits just above the knee
- Green, oversized three-quarter-length coat
- Hip-length, coloured, checked light jacket
- Tailored tweed checked jacket
- Full-length royal blue mac

JOSIE PACKARD

In the pilot, Josie is referred to as 'one of the most beautiful women in the State' and throughout *Twin Peaks* she is frequently seen in designer wear and luxurious fabrics…when Sheriff Truman isn't busy tearing them apart! Josie is so pampered that you can almost smell the expensive perfume through your television set. But underneath all that opulence and wide-eyed innocence, she is a dangerous, ruthless woman and believes any problem can be solved with a bullet.

You needn't have Josie's wallet to have her look; here's a few ideas:

- Red, three-quarter-length, long-sleeved dress
- Elegant white, deep V-neck shirt
- Tailored black jacket

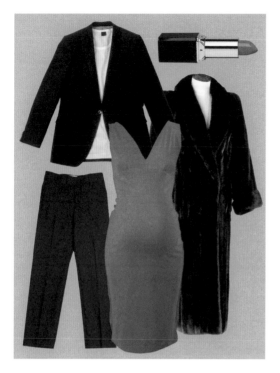

the sweet high school 17 year old who appeared to be every parent's dream. But by night she was fuelled by drugs, sex and self destruction. In her short and desperate life she fought to keep true to herself but was eventually overpowered by the one man who forced his way in.

Here we have chosen a few key items to portray the two lives of Laura Palmer.

- Knee-length checked skirt in brown, green and cream colours
- Green, waist-length, button-up cardigan
- Brown, hip-length knitted jumper
- Green opaque tights
- Black opaque tights
- Brown round-neck T-shirt
- Brown waist-length cardigan
- Flat black pumps

- Long black satin nightgown with side split
- Long black faux-fur coat
- Grey chino-style trousers
- Brown woollen jacket with embroidered hem
- Large green and blue tartan scarf used as a jacket
- Black tailored trousers

LAURA PALMER

So you want to dress like the homecoming queen? Or maybe you prefer the look of Laura's darker and troubled side? There is no doubt that Laura Palmer led an intense double life. By day she was the homecoming queen,

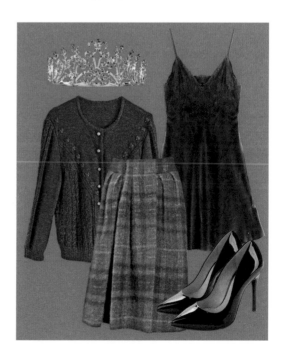

- Above-the-knee black dress, sleeveless with plunging neckline
- Short black tailored jacket
- Long black wrap-around dress with long sleeves
- Short black satin nightdress
- Long black satin nightdress
- Pale pink basque and suspender set
- Black stiletto heels
- Long, olive green woollen coat

BOBBY BRIGGS

He's the town's resident bad boy but we can't help but love Bobby Briggs. That handsome heartbreaker with a charming smile who knows how to appeal to the ladies, Bobby has a very typical high school heart throb look. Think Johnny Depp in *Cry Baby*, and you're halfway there!

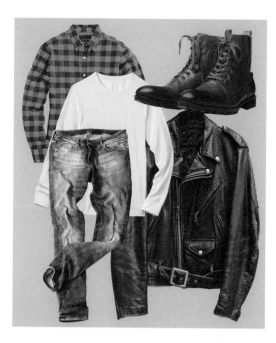

Get Bobby's laid-back cool style with these key items:

- Black leather jacket with granddad collar
- Blue slouch jeans
- Variety of checked shirts sometimes worn round the waist
- Long-sleeved white T-shirt
- Short-sleeved dark red T-shirt
- Short-sleeved bright blue T-shirt
- Blue collared shirt
- Black suit
- Grey, blue and lilac striped tie
- Heavy boots, not fully laced

AGENT COOPER

Entering the town of Twin Peaks at 11.30am on 24 February 1989, Special Agent Dale Cooper brought an air of elegance and sophistication with him. Sheriff Truman says he is the "finest lawman he has ever seen" and Cooper uses cunning, instinct and, dare we say, magic to apprehend the killer of Laura Palmer. And he does all this with a striking sense of style.

Bring out your inner Agent Cooper by filling up your wardrobe with the following:

- Tailored sharp black suit
- Tailored white shirt
- Black, red and white diagonal striped tie
- Black tie with silver diagonal stripes
- Plain black tie

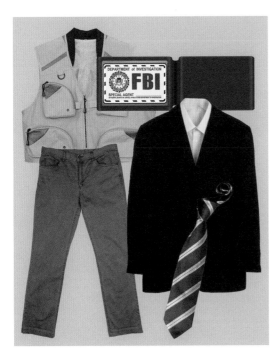

Agent Cooper comes to town to take over the murder case, he welcomes his skill and expertise. Harry is warm and welcoming and this is reflected in his comforting dress sense.

To get cosy like Sheriff Truman, wrap yourself up in these pieces:

- Brown/tan collared shirt
- Black tweed thigh-length jacket (with broken white stripes patterned into squares to be precise!)
- Black V-neck sweater
- Black chunky round-neck jumper
- Ivory chino-style trousers
- Black round-neck T-shirt
- Black padded winter coat
- Black sheriff hat (like a Stetson)
- Gun belt (optional!)

- Long light brown collared mac
- Grey and black checked shirt
- Grey, dark green and red checked shirt
- Olive green trousers
- Royal blue pyjamas, the long-sleeved shirt variety
- Highly polished black shoes
- Leather boots

SHERIFF TRUMAN

If there is one man who takes pride in keeping his town safe, it's Sheriff Harry S. Truman. The murder of Laura Palmer is hard for him to take in a town where a yellow light still means slow down and not speed up. But even he knows there is "evil in those old woods" and when

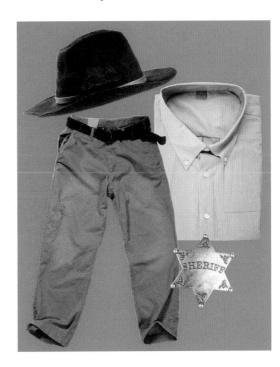

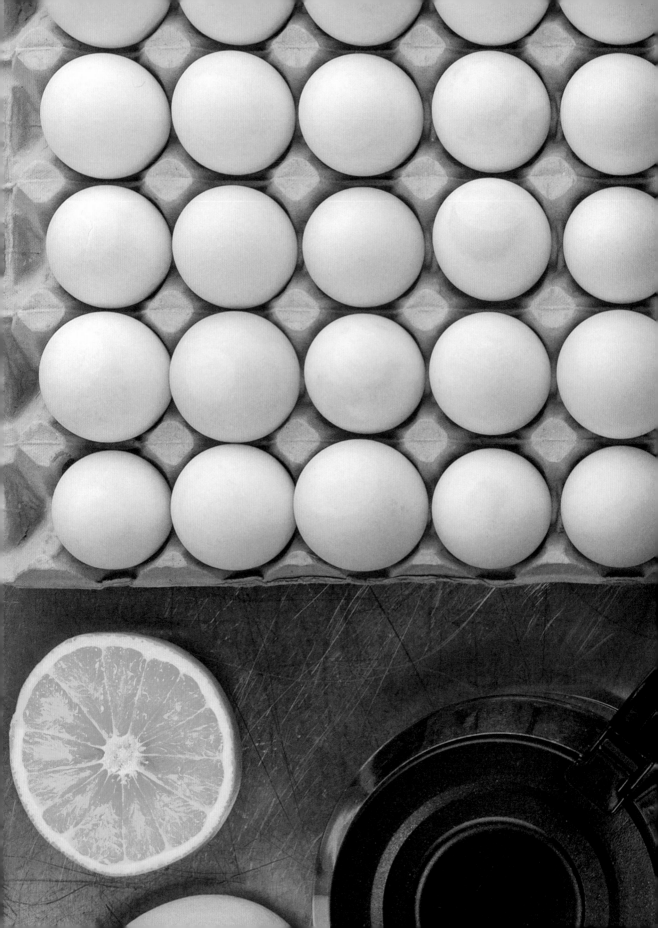

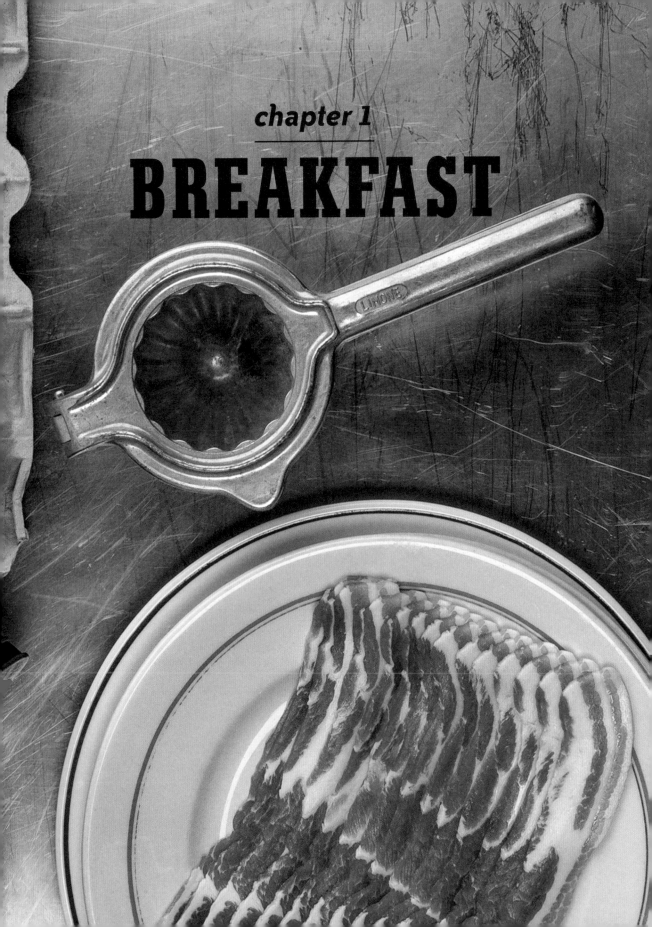

chapter 1

BREAKFAST

BREAKFAST

Breakfast – the most important meal of the day, certainly by Agent Cooper's standards. Whether it's super-crispy bacon, artery-hardening eggs or maple syrup colliding with ham, the man knows what he likes… just as long as it comes with a cup of Great Northern coffee.

Of course, not all *Twin Peaks* residents are as enthusiastic about their morning meal. Bobby Briggs is up at 5am to go running before football practice with just a brief pit-stop at the RR Diner for his morning coffee (or really to share some time with smokin' waitress Shelly Johnson), while Sarah Palmer just has a long smoke with a cup o' Joe. Pete Martell uses his mornings to go fishing rather than eat breakfast… and he has been known to stumble across a homecoming queen wrapped in plastic while other people are enjoying their eggs!

So what better way to start our culinary journey than to delve into the world of good old American breakfasts. This section contains an abundance of delicious food to help you start your day the Agent Dale Cooper way!

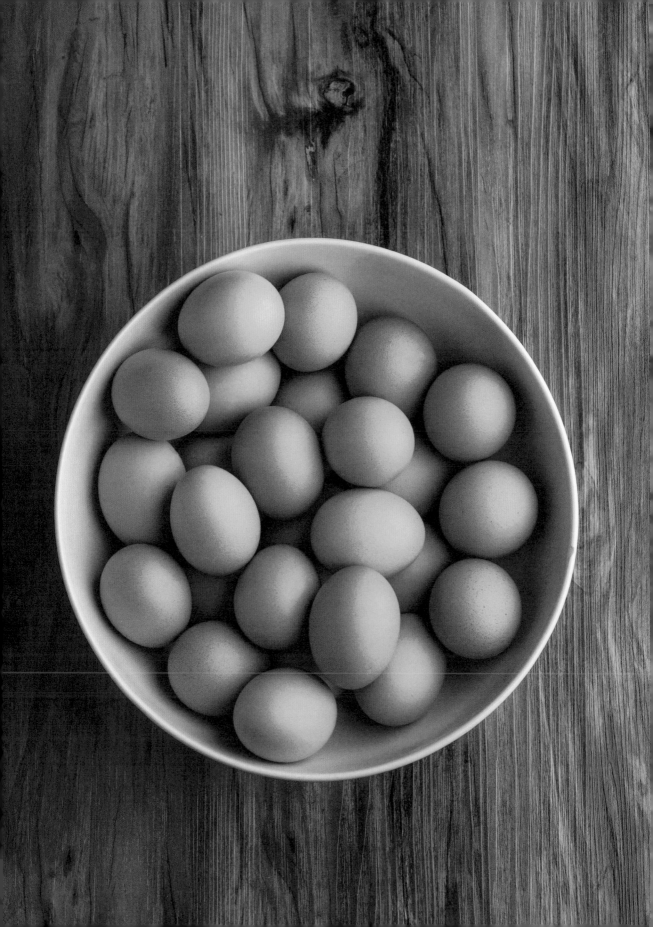

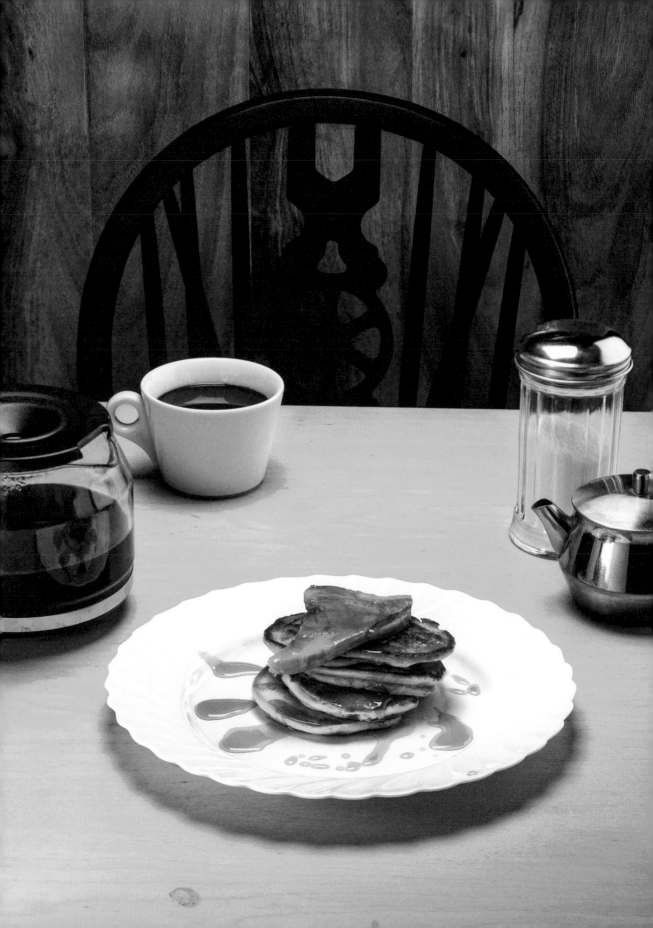

MAPLE HAM PANCAKES

MAKES ABOUT 18 PANCAKES
PREPARATION TIME: 10 MINUTES
COOKING TIME: 25 MINUTES

150g (1¼ cups) plain flour

2 heaped teaspoons baking powder

½ teaspoon bicarbonate of soda

1 teaspoon sugar

pinch of salt

2 eggs

300ml (1¼ cups) milk or buttermilk

100g (7 tablespoons) butter, melted

4 tablespoons maple syrup, plus extra
to serve

200g (7oz) thick-cut, cooked ham slices

❶ Place the flour, baking powder, bicarbonate of soda, sugar and salt in a large bowl. Beat the eggs, milk and half the melted butter together in a jug, then whisk into the dry ingredients until smooth. Set aside.

❷ Place a little of the remaining butter in a large nonstick frying pan over a medium heat, then add a few spoonfuls of the batter mixture. Cook for 2 minutes or until bubbles start to appear on the surface, then flip the pancake and cook for 1–2 minutes on the other side until golden. Remove and keep warm while you cook the remaining pancakes.

❸ Wipe the pan with kitchen paper, then add 3 tablespoons of the maple syrup and put the pan back on the heat. When the syrup is bubbling, slide the ham slices into the pan and cook for 1–2 minutes, turning once or twice, until glazed and sticky. Set aside and keep warm.

❹ Serve a pile of hot pancakes per person topped with the sticky maple ham slices and extra maple syrup on the side.

AGENT COOPER'S SUPER-CRISPY BACON BREAKFAST

TO MAKE CREMATED BACON

1 Line a baking sheet with foil and arrange slices of bacon on it in a single layer.

2 Place on the middle shelf of a cold oven and set the temperature to 200°C (400°F), Gas Mark 6.

3 Check the bacon after 15 minutes, but return to the oven if it isn't quite ready. It should be good and crisp by 20 minutes, but if you want it really cremated then carry on cooking…

4 Drain the bacon on kitchen paper before serving.

For crispy bacon that's still a little chewy

1 Arrange slices of bacon in a single layer in a frying pan.

2 Pour over enough water just to cover the bacon.

3 Place the pan over a medium–high heat and cook for about 5 minutes, turning the bacon once, until the water has boiled off.

4 Lower the heat to medium and cook the bacon for a further 5–8 minutes, turning the slices every now and then, until crispy.

5 Drain the bacon on kitchen paper before serving.

For the eggs

1 Heat a little oil in a heavy-based frying pan over a low–medium heat and break in the eggs, taking care not to break the yolks. Cook according to your preference, as follows:

- **Over Hard** – Cooked on the first side, then flipped over and fried on the other side. The yolk has been broken and is fully cooked.

- **Over Well** – Cooked on the first side, then flipped over and fried on the other side. The unbroken yolk is fully cooked.

- **Over Medium Well** – Cooked on the first side, then flipped over and lightly fried on the other side. The unbroken yolk is cooked, but still a little soft in the centre.

- **Over Medium** – Cooked on the first side, then flipped over and lightly fried on the other side. The whites are fully cooked, but the unbroken yolk is still runny.

- **Over Easy** – Cooked on the first side, then flipped over and very lightly fried on the other side. The whites are not fully cooked, and the unbroken yolk is runny.

- **Basted Sunny-side Up** – Cooked on one side only. Hot fat is spooned over the white and yolk while the egg is cooking, so the yolk becomes opaque but is still a little runny.

- **Sunny-side Up** – Cooked briefly on one side only. The yolk is still liquid and whites a little runny.

GORDON COLE'S SMALL MEXICAN BREAKFAST BURRITOS

SERVES 4
PREPARATION TIME: 40 MINUTES
COOKING TIME: 1 HOUR

12 soft corn or wheat tortillas

handful of fresh coriander leaves

200ml (scant 1 cup) soured cream

100g (1 cup) hard white cheese, crumbled

1 large avocado, peeled, pitted and sliced

salt and pepper

4 lime wedges, to serve

Refried beans

3 tablespoons olive oil

75g (1/3 cup) smoked streaky bacon, chopped, or smoked bacon lardons

1 onion, finely chopped

2 garlic cloves, crushed

1–2 jalapeño chillies, deseeded and chopped

pinch of ground cumin

2 x 400-g (14-oz) cans pinto, black or kidney beans, rinsed and drained

Salsa ranchera

3 tablespoons olive oil

½ red onion, finely chopped

1 garlic clove, finely chopped

1 red chilli, deseeded and finely chopped

400g (2 cups) ripe tomatoes, chopped

Mushrooms

3 tablespoons olive oil

200g (2²/3 cups) Portobello mushrooms, finely sliced

¼ teaspoon smoked paprika

Scrambled egg

3 eggs, lightly beaten

3 tablespoons soured cream or crème fraîche

25g (2 tablespoons) butter

❶ For the refried beans, heat the oil in a large heavy-based saucepan, add the bacon and cook, stirring occasionally, until golden. Add the onion, garlic, jalapeños and cumin and cook for 5–6 minutes until softened.

❷ Stir in the drained beans and mash half of them with a potato masher or fork. Stir in a little water. Season and cook for a few minutes, adding more liquid if necessary, until you have a thick purée.

❸ To make the salsa, place the oil in a large saucepan, add the onion and garlic and cook for 5–6 minutes or until softened. Add the chilli and continue to cook for another minute before adding the tomatoes. Bring to the boil, reduce the heat and simmer for about 20 minutes or until thickened. Season to taste.

❹ When ready to serve, warm the tortillas one at a time in a dry frying pan. Wrap in a tea towel to keep warm while you heat the rest.

❺ For the mushrooms, heat the oil in a large frying pan over a medium heat, add the mushrooms and season with salt, pepper and smoked paprika. Cook for 3–4 minutes, stirring occasionally, until the mushrooms are tender.

❻ Place the eggs in a bowl with the soured cream, season and beat together lightly. Place the butter in a small pan over a medium heat and when it's foaming, pour in the egg mixture. Let it sit for a moment or two, then stir quickly and scramble until soft but just holding its shape.

❼ Place the coriander leaves, soured cream, white cheese, sliced avocado and lime wedges into separate bowls. Serve the warm tortillas with all the other components so everyone can build their own burritos.

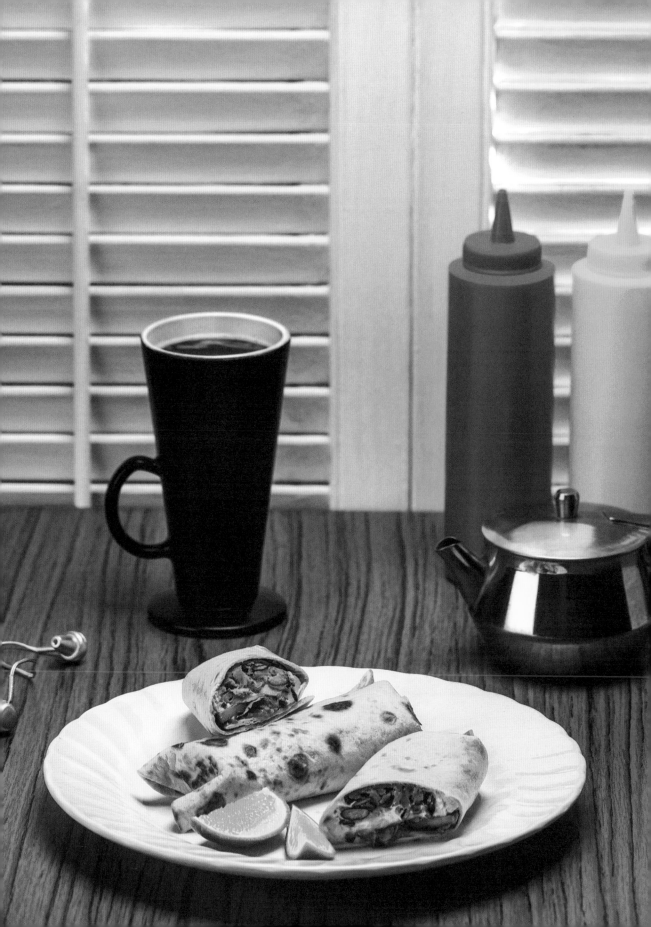

LEO JOHNSON'S STEAK & EGG SANDWICH

SERVES 4
PREPARATION TIME: 20 MINUTES
COOKING TIME: 50 MINUTES

4 large Portobello or field mushrooms

4 tablespoons olive oil

50g (3½ tablespoons) butter

4 x 225-g (8-oz) sirloin, rump or bavette steaks

200ml (scant 1 cup) water

8 slices of crusty bread, toasted

handful of baby spinach

salt and pepper

Slow-cooked onions

6 tablespoons olive oil

2 teaspoons mustard seeds

2 large red onions, thinly sliced

2 garlic cloves, crushed

4 tablespoons chopped flat-leaf parsley

1 tablespoon balsamic vinegar

Fried eggs

2 tablespoons olive oil

50g (3½ tablespoons) butter

2 tablespoons sage leaves

4 eggs

❶ For the onions, heat the olive oil in a frying pan over a medium heat, add the mustard seeds and let them pop for 30 seconds (do not let them burn). Add the onions and garlic, reduce the heat, cover and cook gently without browning for 30 minutes until very soft. Stir in the parsley and vinegar, season and set aside.

❷ Meanwhile, brush the mushrooms with half the olive oil, season. Preheat a grill to high and cook for 5–8 minutes, turning occasionally, until tender. Season the steaks.

❸ Place the remaining oil and the butter in a large frying pan over a medium heat and heat until the butter is foaming and light brown (don't let it burn). Raise the heat to medium–high, lay the steaks in the foaming butter and cook for 1½–2 minutes on each side for rare, 3 minutes for medium-rare, or 4 minutes for medium. Transfer the steaks to a warm plate to rest. Return the pan to the heat, add the measured water, scraping the bottom of the pan with a wooden spoon, and let it sizzle until thickened.

❹ For the eggs, heat the oil and butter in a clean frying pan until foaming, then slide in the sage leaves. Carefully break the eggs into the pan and fry until cooked to your liking.

❺ Meanwhile, place a slice of toast on each of 4 serving plates and arrange a handful of spinach leaves on each. Top with a cooked mushroom and spoon some of the onions into each one. Slice the steak and divide between the sandwiches, then top with a fried egg, sage leaves and some of the cooking juices. Top with another slice of toast and serve immediately.

J'AI UNE ÂME SOLITAIRE FRENCH TOAST

SERVES 4
PREPARATION TIME: 5 MINUTES
COOKING TIME: 8–12 MINUTES

3 eggs

50ml (scant ¼ cup) milk

½ teaspoon ground cinnamon

25g (2 tablespoons) butter

8 slices of raisin and cinnamon bread

8 tablespoons demerara or cinnamon sugar

4 scoops of ice cream or frozen yogurt,
to serve (optional)

1 Place the eggs, milk and cinnamon in a large, shallow bowl and beat until well combined. Melt half the butter in a large, nonstick frying pan over a medium heat.

2 Dip 4 slices of the bread in the egg mixture and sprinkle both sides with half the sugar.

3 Place the coated bread in the pan of melted butter and cook gently for 4–6 minutes, turning once, until golden and crispy. Drain on kitchen paper and keep warm. Repeat the process with the remaining slices of bread. Serve with ice cream or frozen yogurt, if desired.

JOHNNY HORNE'S TOTEM TOWER

SERVES 6
PREPARATION TIME: 1½ HOURS,
PLUS RISING
COOKING TIME: ABOUT 1 HOUR

50g (1 cup) fresh white breadcrumbs

100ml (scant ½ cup) milk

600g (scant 3 cups) minced pork

100g (scant ½ cup) canned sweetcorn, drained

50g (½ cup) Parmesan cheese, finely grated

handful of flat-leaf parsley, finely chopped

finely grated zest of 1 lemon

1 teaspoon fennel seeds, crushed

2 tablespoons thyme leaves

1 egg, beaten

flour, for dusting

3 tablespoons olive oil

3 beef tomatoes, thickly sliced

12 smoked bacon rashers dry-fried
until crisp

salt and pepper

English muffins

450g (3½ cups) plain flour, plus extra
for dusting

50g (3½ tablespoons) butter, plus extra
for greasing

3 teaspoons fast-action dried yeast

2 teaspoons caster sugar

250ml (1 generous cup) milk

fine cornmeal or polenta, for sprinkling

Relish

6 jalapeño chillies

1 large onion, peeled and quartered

2 garlic cloves

3 tablespoons olive oil

1 large avocado, peeled and pitted

juice of 1 lime

4 tablespoons fresh coriander,
finely chopped

❶ For the English muffins, place the flour in a bowl, add the butter and rub in with the fingertips until the mixture resembles fine breadcrumbs. Stir in the yeast and sugar, then stir in the milk with a fork, then your fingers, and bring the mixture together to form a soft dough. Turn out on to a lightly floured surface and knead for about 10 minutes or until smooth and elastic. Transfer to a greased bowl, cover and set aside for about 1 hour or until doubled in size.

❷ Knock back the dough and roll out on a lightly floured surface to about 1cm (½ inch) thick. Cut out rounds with a 8-cm (3¼-inch) straight-sided cutter, reroll the trimmings and cut out more muffins, giving 12 in total. Lightly sprinkle 2 baking sheets with cornmeal and arrange the muffins on the sheets. Dust a little more cornmeal over the tops. Set aside for 30 minutes until puffy. Preheat a heavy-based frying pan over a low heat, sprinkle it with cornmeal and cook the muffins in batches for 4–5 minutes on each side until golden. Cool on a wire rack.

❸ For the relish, preheat the oven to 200°C (400°F), Gas Mark 6, place the chillies, onion and garlic in an ovenproof dish and toss with the oil and a pinch of salt. Cover with foil and cook for 35–45 minutes or until very soft. Leave to cool. Peel and mash the garlic, destalk the chillies (removing seeds if liked), and chop with the onion. Scrape the mixture into a bowl and mash in the avocado. Stir in the lime juice and coriander and season.

❹ Place the breadcrumbs in a bowl, add the milk and soak for 10 minutes. Squeeze out the excess milk and transfer the breadcrumbs to a large bowl with the pork, sweetcorn, Parmesan, parsley, lemon zest, fennel seeds, thyme and egg. Season and combine. Shape into 12 flat patties, each about 1½cm (5/8in) thick, and dust with flour. Heat a little oil in a large nonstick frying pan over a medium heat. Cook the patties in batches for 4–5 minutes on each side until cooked through.

❺ Split and toast the muffins. To make a tower, place the base of a muffin on a plate then layer the relish, tomatoes, patties and bacon as shown in the photograph. Finally, place a muffin lid on top. Repeat to make 6 towers and serve immediately.

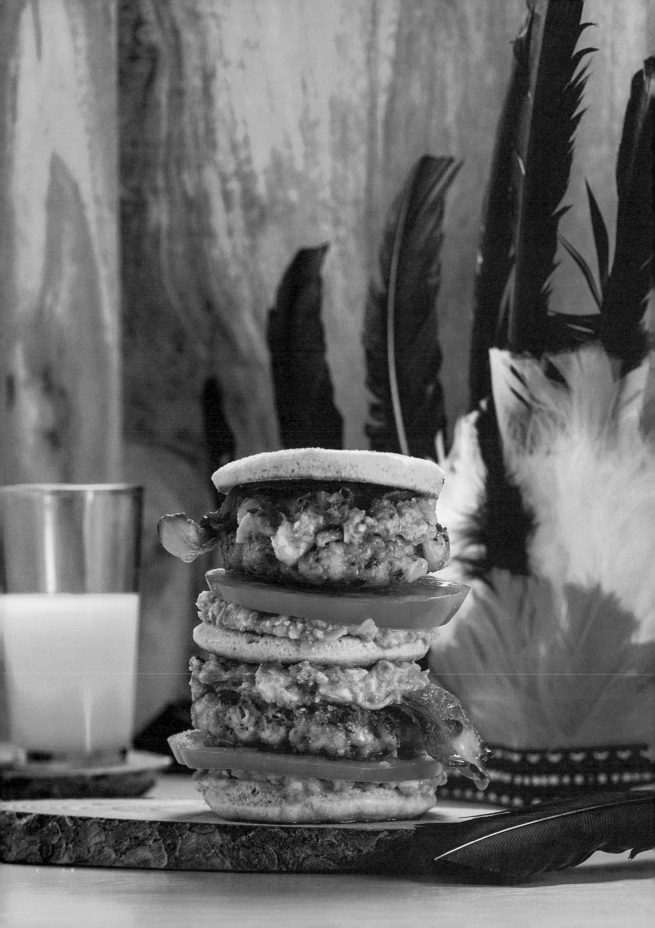

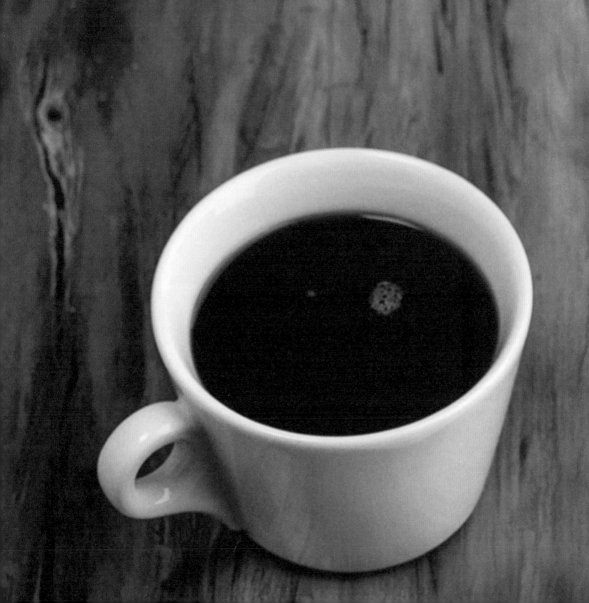

The world consumes close to 2.25 billion cups of coffee every day. Caffeine has most impact on the body between 9.30 and 11.30 in the morning – the perfect time for a Great Northern breakfast!

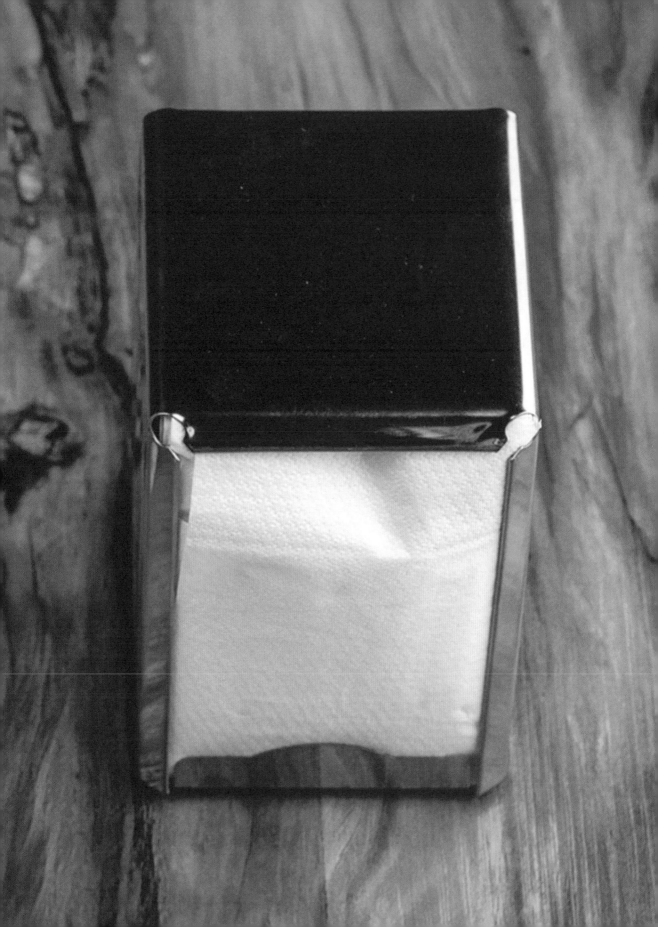

THE OWLS ARE NOT WHAT THEY SEEM

Origami owls make effective *Twin Peaks* theme decorations. You could also challenge your guests to make their own owl at a dinner party inspired by *Twin Peaks*. Who can do it in the shortest time?

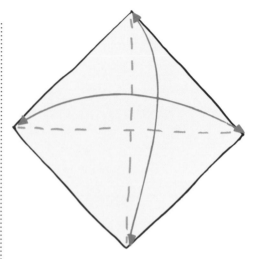

1 Start with a square piece of paper, preferably coloured on one side, white on the other. With the coloured side up, fold the paper in half diagonally, then open it again. Fold it in half diagonally the other way and open it again.

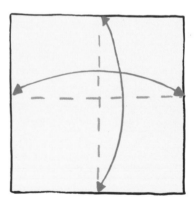

2 Turn the paper over so the white side is facing up. Fold the paper in half horizontally, crease well and open, and then fold in half again in the other direction and open.

3 Using the creases you have made, bring the top three points of the model down to the bottom point and flatten the model into a square.

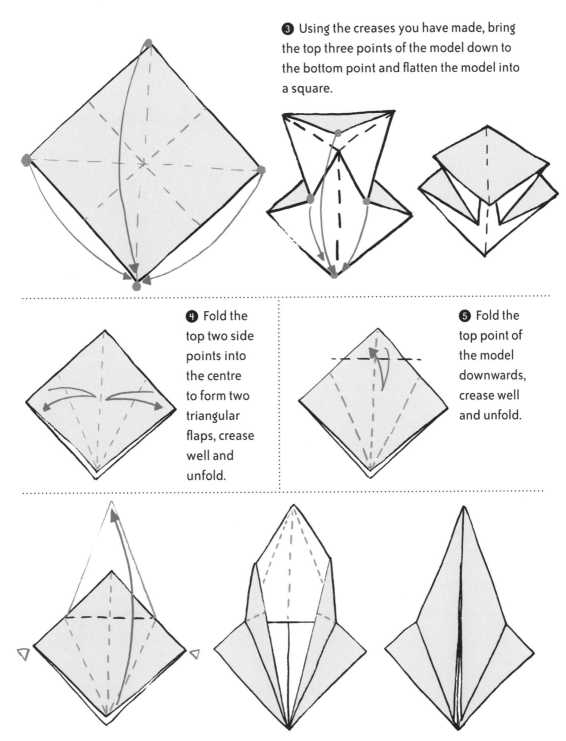

4 Fold the top two side points into the centre to form two triangular flaps, crease well and unfold.

5 Fold the top point of the model downwards, crease well and unfold.

6 From the bottom point, lift the top layer of the model and bring it upwards, pressing the sides of the model inwards at the same time. Flatten down to crease well.

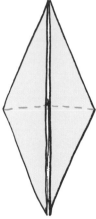

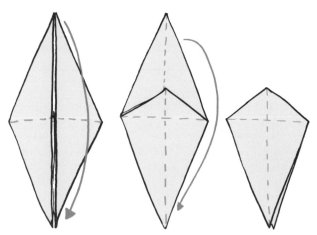

7 Turn over and repeat steps 4, 5 and 6 on the other side of the model.

8 Fold the top point down to meet the bottom, on first the front and then the back of the model.

9 On the top layer, fold the two side points into the centre line, then turn the model over and repeat.

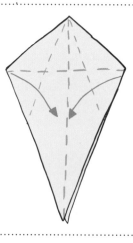

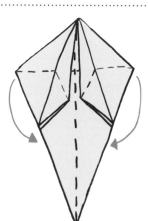

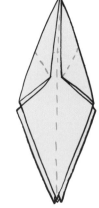

10 Make the wings by pulling out the inner flap from each side and twisting it forwards, then squashing down.

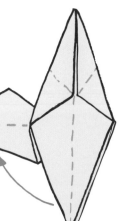

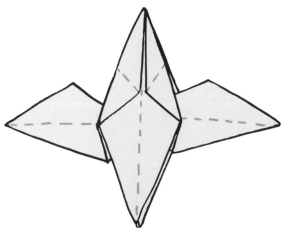

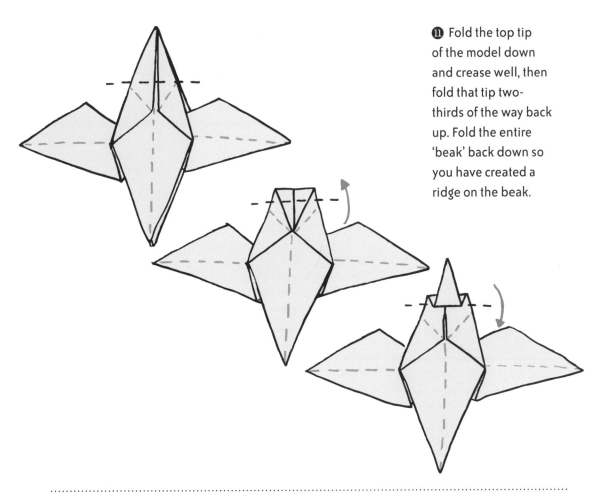

11 Fold the top tip of the model down and crease well, then fold that tip two-thirds of the way back up. Fold the entire 'beak' back down so you have created a ridge on the beak.

12 Finally, use a permanent marker to give your owl eyes to watch you!

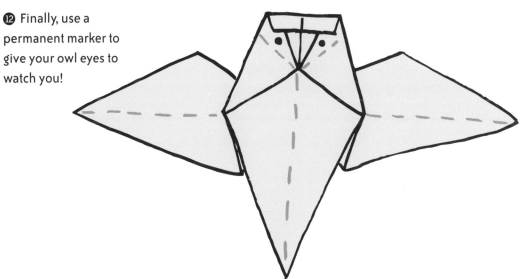

PARMESAN EGG BREAD

SERVES 6
PREPARATION TIME: 10 MINUTES
COOKING TIME: 8–14 MINUTES

6 plum tomatoes

4 tablespoons ready-made olive tapenade

extra virgin olive oil, for drizzling

150ml (⅔ cup) milk

3 eggs

3 tablespoons freshly grated Parmesan cheese

50g (3½ tablespoons) butter

6 slices of white bread

handful of baby spinach leaves

salt and pepper

a few basil leaves, to garnish

❶ Preheat the grill to hot. Cut the tomatoes in half and scoop out the seeds. Arrange them, cut-side up, in a baking dish. Spoon a little of the tapenade on to each tomato and drizzle with some oil. Grill for 2–3 minutes until soft and golden. Keep warm.

❷ Place the milk, eggs, Parmesan and a little salt and pepper in a large, shallow bowl and beat until combined. Melt half the butter in a large, nonstick frying pan over a medium heat.

❸ Dip 3 slices of the bread in the egg mixture. Place the coated bread in the pan of melted butter and cook gently for 4–6 minutes, turning once, until golden and crispy. Drain on kitchen paper and keep warm. Repeat the process with the remaining slices of bread.

❹ Serve the eggy bread topped with the grilled tomatoes and baby spinach leaves, garnished with a few basil leaves.

GREAT NORTHERN HOTEL
BANANA CINNAMON OATMEAL

SERVES 4
PREPARATION TIME: 5 MINUTES
COOKING TIME: 10–15 MINUTES

150g (scant 2 cups) porridge oats

300ml (1¼ cups) milk

600ml (2½ cups) boiling water

2 bananas

4 tablespoons light or dark muscovado sugar

¼ teaspoon ground cinnamon

1 Place the oats, milk and measured boiling water in a heavy-based saucepan over a medium heat. Bring to the boil, stirring, then reduce the heat and simmer for 5–6 minutes, stirring frequently, until the oats are soft and the mixture is thick and creamy.

2 Spoon the oatmeal into bowls, then slice the bananas and arrange on top. Mix together the sugar and cinnamon and sprinkle over the bananas. Serve immediately.

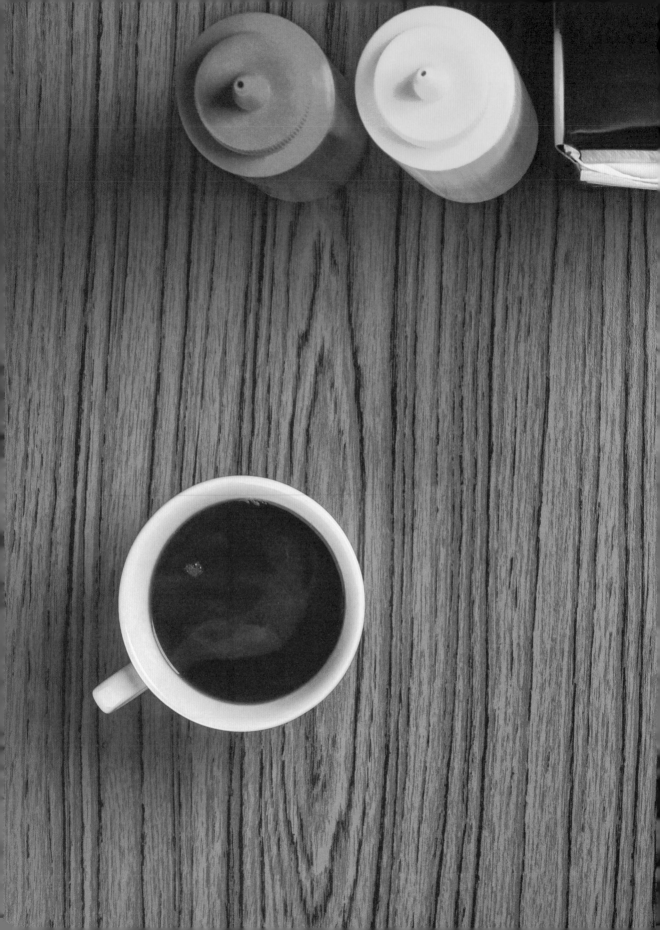

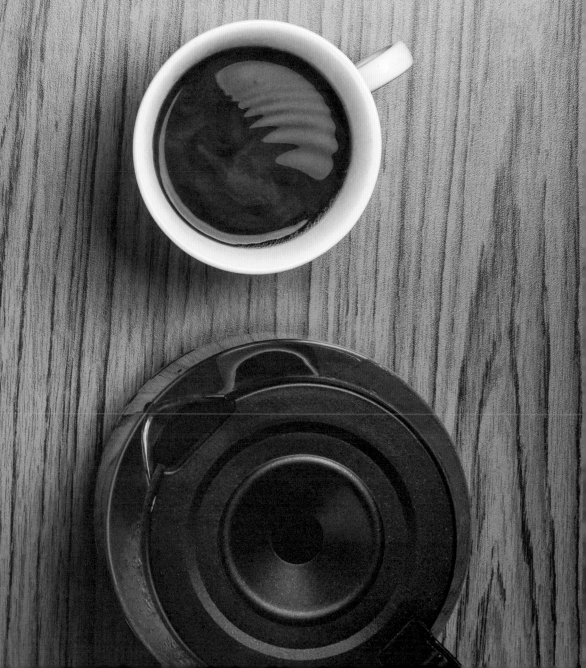

chapter 2

DINER MENU

DINER

Surely the backbone of the town of *Twin Peaks* must be the RR Diner. Where else would you meet your fellow townsfolk for a damn fine cup of coffee and catch up on the latest murder? In fact, half of the main characters in the show are seen in the RR at least once and it has played host to scenes of humour, heartbreak, cunning, violence, flirting, fear and waitresses who can't get their cars started.

So many famous and well-written scenes take place in the diner. From Agent Cooper's declaration that you should give yourself a daily gift of coffee to the poignant moment when Major Briggs shares his beautiful dream about his son. Scenes like these give the show its charm and depth.

The RR Diner is seen as a safe place for the townsfolk, especially for owner Norma Jennings and her trusty sidekick Shelly Johnson. Shelly is sadly a victim of domestic abuse at the hands of her husband Leo Johnson. But what she loses in love for her husband she makes up for with a passionate affair with bad boy Bobby Briggs. And there is more passion at the RR Diner as Norma carries on an affair with her former flame 'Big Ed' Hurley, while her husband Hank serves three-to-five years for manslaughter.

And of course it would not be the RR without the coffee! As Audrey Horne would tell you, Agent Cooper loves coffee, but coffee is nectar for most of the residents of the town. This of course comes from *Twin Peaks* co-creator David Lynch. It is well known that the man is mad about his coffee, which is why it features heavily in a lot of his work. Did you know that he even has his own brand of coffee: David Lynch Signature Cup Coffee (available from www.twinpeaksukfest.com).

As most Peakies will know, the real RR Diner is Twede's Café in North Bend, Washington. It opened in 1941 as Thompson's Diner and was known as the Mar-T-Café during the filming of *Twin Peaks*. It was bought by current owner Kyle Twede in the late 1990s and has recently seen a fantastic refurbishment by David Lynch's team to return it to its 1989 look. The RR Diner is once again ready to be the backbone of the town in the new season!

I have taken inspiration from my favourite *Twin Peaks* characters and blended them with American diner classics to create a real mix of RR Diner-themed treats. So just pour yourself a cup of **"Good Morning America"** and get cooking!

DR JACOBY'S HAWAIIAN BURGER

SERVES 4
PREPARATION TIME: 20 MINUTES
COOKING TIME: 20–25 MINUTES

1kg (scant 4½ cups) coarsely minced beef

75g (1½ cups) fresh breadcrumbs

6 spring onions, finely chopped

salt and pepper

Avocado and jalapeño cream

1 large avocado, peeled and pitted

1 jalapeño chilli, deseeded

1 tablespoon chopped fresh coriander

finely grated zest and juice of 1 lime

200ml (scant 1 cup) crème fraîche

Caramelized pineapple

25g (2 tablespoons) butter

1 teaspoon brown sugar

¼ teaspoon Chinese five-spice powder
(optional)

4 slices of fresh pineapple, peeled and
core removed

To serve

8 streaky bacon rashers

4 slices of Cheddar cheese

4 soft burger buns, split and toasted

soft lettuce leaves

teriyaki sauce, for drizzling

4 spiky leaves from the top of the pineapple

❶ Lightly mix the minced beef with the breadcrumbs and spring onions and season with salt and pepper. Shape into four patties, 2–3cm (¾–1¼ inches) thick.

❷ For the avocado and jalapeño cream, place the avocado, chilli, coriander and lime zest and juice in a food processor and blend until smooth. Scrape into a bowl, stir in the crème fraîche and season to taste.

❸ For the caramelized pineapple, melt the butter in a heavy-based frying pan over a medium heat. Add the sugar and five-spice, if using, then slide in the pineapple slices and cook for 3–4 minutes, turning once, or until lightly browned on both sides. Remove from the pan and set aside, then add the bacon and fry until crispy.

❹ Preheat a grill or griddle pan to medium–high and cook the patties for 4–5 minutes per side for rare to medium, or 8–10 minutes for medium to well done. Lay a slice of Cheddar on top of each burger during the last minute of cooking to soften.

❺ Lay the bases of the toasted buns on 4 serving plates, top with lettuce, the patties, a splash of teriyaki sauce, a spoonful of avocado and jalapeño cream, a slice of pineapple and 2 bacon rashers. Place the bun lids on the burgers and use spikes from the pineapple top to pin the ingredients together.

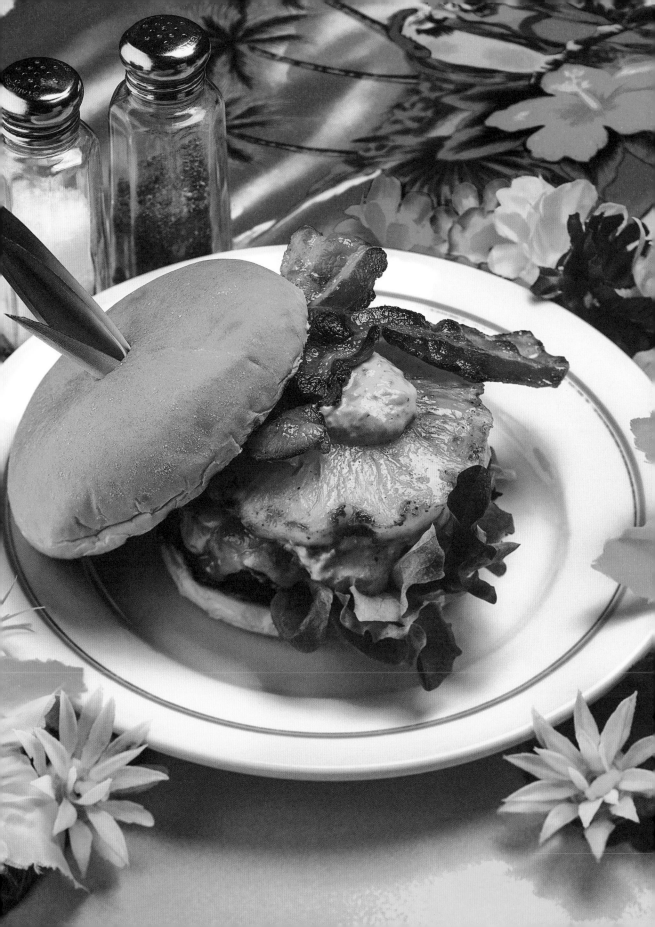

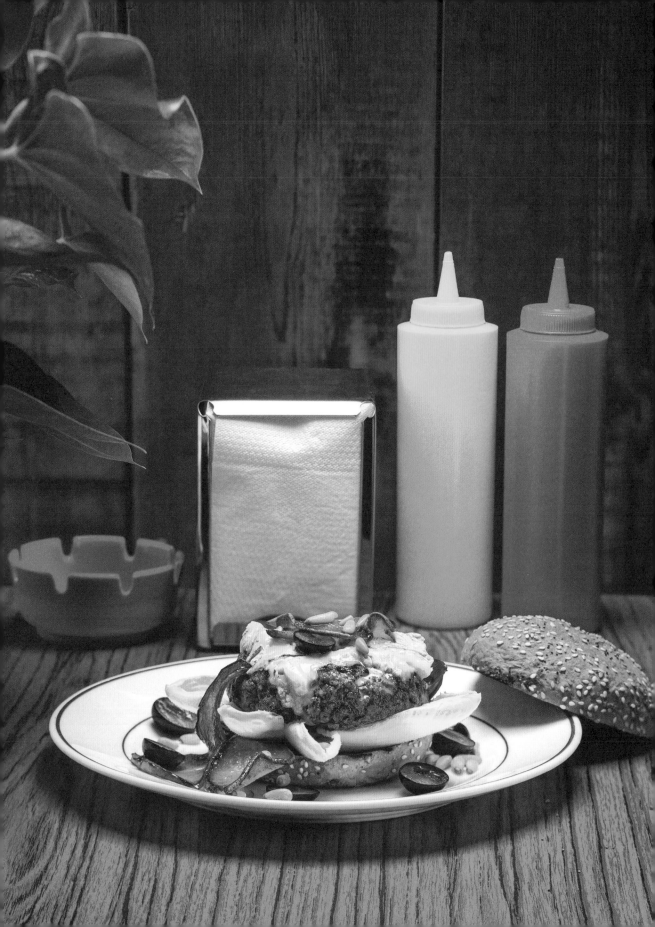

MOUNTAIN HARLEY BURGER

SERVES 4
PREPARATION TIME: 30 MINUTES
COOKING TIME: 20 MINUTES

1kg (scant 4½ cups) coarsely minced beef
75g (1½ cups) fresh breadcrumbs
6 spring onions, finely chopped
salt and pepper

Caramelized pears

25g (2 tablespoons) unsalted butter
2 teaspoons soft brown sugar
2 pears, cored and thickly sliced
1 tablespoon red wine vinegar

To serve

4 burger buns, warmed and split
4 thick slices of Gorgonzola dolce or other blue cheese (about 200g/7oz in total)
1 head of chicory, leaves separated
50g (5 tablespoons) pine nuts or pecans, toasted
100g (1 cup) black grapes, halved, deseeded and chilled

① Lightly mix the minced beef with the breadcrumbs and spring onions and season with salt and pepper. Shape into 4 patties, 2–3cm (¾–1¼ inches) thick.

② For the caramelized pears, melt the butter in a large frying pan over a medium–high heat, sprinkle in the sugar, add the pears and cook for 2–3 minutes on each side until golden and slightly caramelized. Add the red wine vinegar, swirl around the pan, remove from the heat and set aside.

③ Preheat a grill or griddle pan to medium–high and lightly toast the burger buns and set aside. Now cook the patties for 4–5 minutes per side for rare to medium, or 8–10 minutes for medium to well done. Lay a slice of Gorgonzola on top of each burger during the last minute of cooking to soften.

④ Lay the bases of the warmed buns on 4 serving plates, top with chicory leaves, add a few slices of caramelized pear and then the patties. Scatter with toasted pine nuts, chilled grapes and another couple of slices of pear, then top with the bun lids and serve.

James Marshall, who portrayed the character of James Hurley, really does play the guitar and really did sing the song 'Just You' in *Twin Peaks*.

POUTINE WITH RED-EYE GRAVY

SERVES 4
PREPARATION TIME: 30 MINUTES
COOKING TIME: 30 MINUTES

1kg (2lb 4oz) floury potatoes

2 litres (8½ cups) groundnut, corn or sunflower oil, for deep-frying, or 4 tablespoons for oven baking

sea salt flakes

soft cheese curds, to serve

Red-eye gravy

50g (3½ tablespoons) butter

300g (10½oz) gammon steaks, cut into strips

1 onion, finely chopped

1 garlic clove, crushed

a few thyme sprigs

400ml (1⅔ cups) strong black espresso coffee

400ml (1⅔ cups) beef stock

1 teaspoon light brown sugar

2 tablespoons cornflour mixed with 4 tablespoons water

salt and pepper

❶ For the gravy, melt the butter in a heavy-based frying pan over a medium heat. When it starts to foam, add the gammon strips and cook, stirring occasionally, for 3–4 minutes until well browned. Add the onion, garlic and thyme and cook for a further 3–4 minutes until softened. Season to taste.

❷ Pour in the coffee and let it bubble up and deglaze the pan, scraping the base of the pan with a wooden spoon to loosen any residue. Add the stock and sugar and bring to the boil. Add the cornflour mixture and stir until thickened. Strain into a jug.

❸ Cut the potatoes into 5-mm (¼-inch) slices, leaving the skin on. Cut the slices into 5-mm (¼-inch) fries, rinse thoroughly in cold water to remove surface starch and drain well. Pat the fries with a clean tea towel, transfer to another clean dry tea towel and dry again.

❹ Pour the oil into a large, deep saucepan or deep-fat fryer, making sure it is no more than one-third to one-half full. Heat the oil until it reaches 160°C (325°F). Carefully lower the fries, in batches, into the hot oil and cook for 5 minutes until tender but still pale. Drain well on kitchen paper.

❺ Raise the heat of the oil to 190°C (375°F) and carefully lower the blanched fries back into the oil, again in batches. Cook for 1–2 minutes until golden brown and crisp. Drain well on kitchen paper.

❻ Alternatively, to oven bake the fries, preheat the oven to 220°C (425°F), Gas Mark 7. Place the fries with 4 tablespoons of oil in a large bowl and toss to coat, then arrange them in a single layer on 2 baking sheets. Cook for about 30 minutes, shaking the trays and turning the fries occasionally, until golden and crispy. Drain well on kitchen paper.

❼ Tip the fries into a bowl, season with salt and toss well to coat. Transfer to a serving dish, sprinkle with the cheese curds and pour over the gravy. Serve immediately.

See photograph overleaf.

SWEET POTATO MAPLE SYRUP FRIES

SERVES 4
PREPARATION TIME: 20 MINUTES
COOKING TIME: 20 MINUTES

2 large sweet potatoes, peeled
potato or rice flour, for dusting
25g (2 tablespoons) butter
100ml (scant ½ cup) maple syrup
finely grated zest and juice of 2 limes
groundnut or vegetable oil, for deep-frying
sea salt flakes

❶ Cut the sweet potatoes into 5-mm (¼-inch) slices, then cut the slices into 5-mm (¼-inch) fries. Place in a bowl and toss with potato or rice flour, to coat them evenly.

❷ Place the butter, maple syrup and lime zest in a small saucepan over a medium heat. Bring to the boil, lower the heat and simmer for a few minutes until reduced and slightly thickened. Remove from the heat, stir in the lime juice and set aside.

❸ Pour the oil into a large, deep saucepan or deep-fat fryer, making sure it is no more than one-third to one-half full. Heat the oil until it reaches 180°C (350°F). Carefully lower the fries, in batches, into the hot oil and cook for 5–7 minutes until tender and crisp.

❹ Drain the fries on kitchen paper, toss with sea salt flakes and serve drizzled with the maple syrup glaze.

See photograph overleaf.

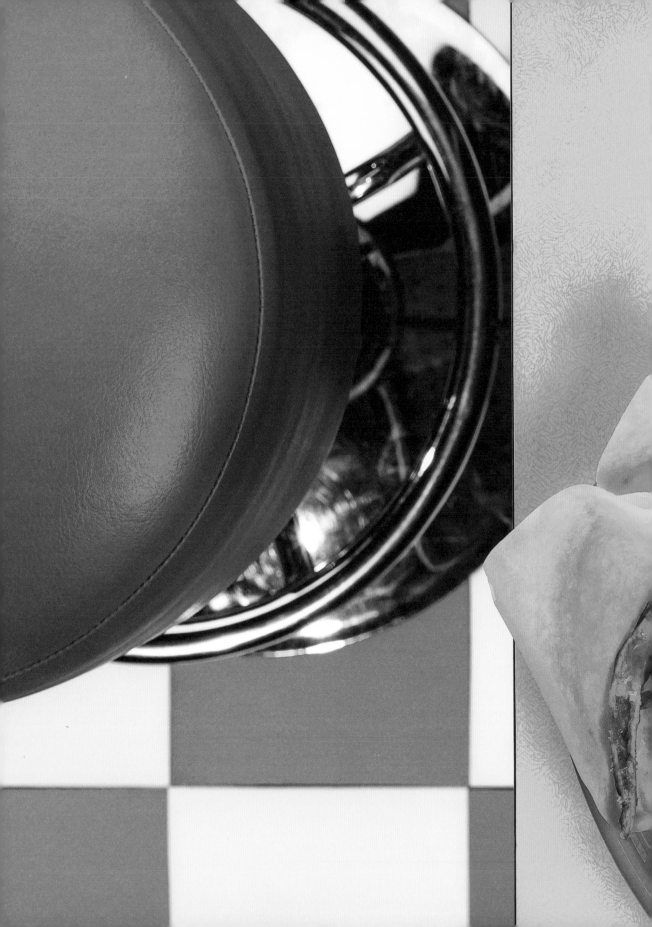

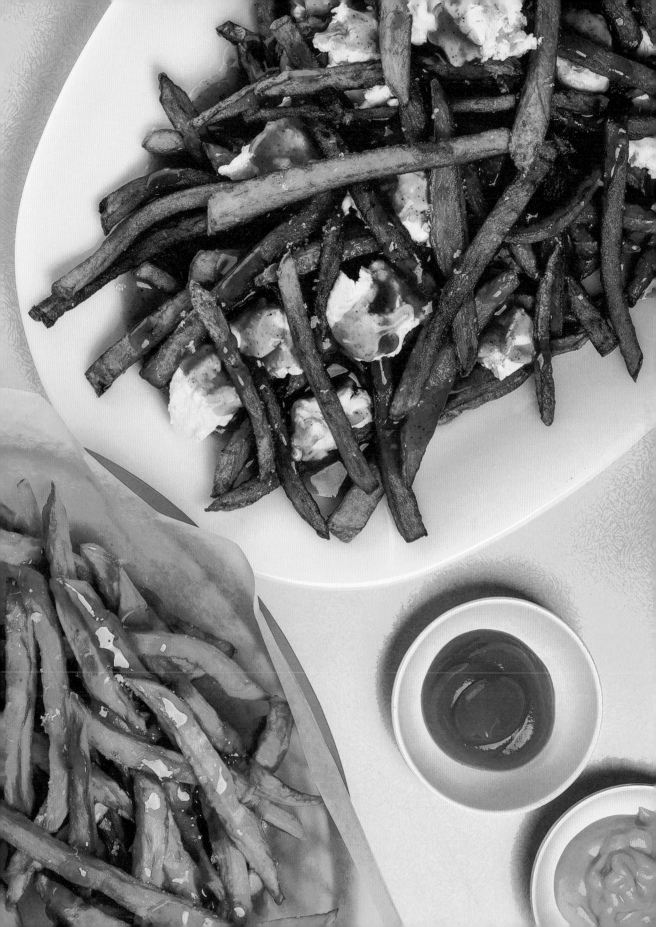

DINER JUKEBOX SELECTION

There's no better way to enhance your Diner experience than by listening to some of the best 50s and 60s music. David Lynch is known for his use of the sounds from this era in his work, so here's an inspired selection for your cooking pleasure.

1   Linda Scott – "I've Told Every Little Star"

2   Bobby Vinton – "Blue Velvet"

3   Sonny Boy Williamson II – "Bring It On Home"

4   Roy Orbison – "In Dreams"

5   Van Morrison and Them – "Baby, Please Don't Go"

6   Gene Vincent and His Blue Caps – "Be-Bop-A-Lula"

7   Elvis Presley – "Love Me Tender"

8   Connie Stevens – "Sixteen Reasons"

9   Frankie Avalon – "Venus"

10 Tommy James and The Shondells – "Crimson and Clover"

11 Connie Francis – "Everybody's Somebody's Fool"

12 Brenda Lee – "All Alone Am I"

13 Bobby Darin – "Dream Lover"

14 Buddy Holly – "That'll Be The Day"

15 Doris Day – "Whatever Will Be, Will Be"

16 The Crew-Cuts – "Sh-Boom"

17 Peggy Lee – "Fever"

18 The Everly Brothers – "Bye Bye Love"

19 Dion and The Belmonts – "A Teenager in Love"

20 Andy Williams – "Moon River"

21 Bobby Vinton – "Roses Are Red (My Love)"

22 Patsy Cline – "Crazy"

23 The Coasters – "Poison Ivy"

24 Danny and The Juniors – "At The Hop"

25 Ray Charles – "I've Got A Woman"

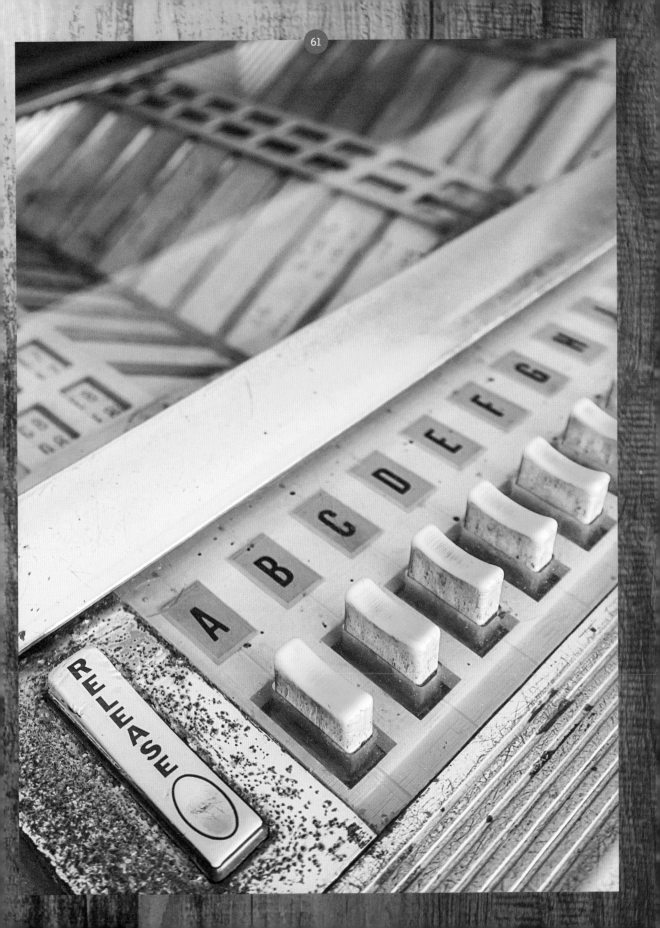

HOT PEANUT BUTTER & JELLY BURGER

SERVES 4
PREPARATION TIME: 30 MINUTES
COOKING TIME: 1 HOUR

1kg (scant 4½ cups) coarsely minced beef

75g (1½ cups) fresh breadcrumbs

salt and pepper

Bacon jam

250g (generous 1 cup) streaky bacon, cut into 1.5-cm (⅝-inch) pieces

3 large shallots, finely sliced

2 garlic cloves, chopped

1 teaspoon dried chilli flakes

1 apple, peeled, cored and chopped

3 tablespoons apple cider vinegar

3 tablespoons maple syrup

3 tablespoons light soft brown sugar

3 tablespoons strong coffee

3 tablespoons bourbon whiskey

Peanut butter mayonnaise

3 egg yolks

1 red chilli, deseeded and finely chopped

1 garlic clove, chopped

2 tablespoons peanut butter

2 tablespoons lemon or lime juice

250ml (generous 1 cup) light olive oil or vegetable oil

To serve

4 burger buns, split and toasted

sliced ripe tomatoes

soft lettuce leaves

1 For the bacon jam, place the bacon in a large dry frying pan and cook over a medium heat for 15–20 minutes, stirring frequently, until golden and crispy. Drain the bacon in a sieve over a bowl then on kitchen paper. Pour 1 tablespoon of the fat back into the pan.

2 Add the shallots to the frying pan with the garlic and chilli flakes and cook over a medium heat for 5 minutes or until softened. Add the remaining jam ingredients, bring the mixture to the boil, lower the heat and simmer, stirring occasionally, for 15–20 minutes or until the liquid reduces to a thick glaze. Cool slightly, then blend to a chunky paste in a food processor.

3 For the peanut butter mayonnaise, place the egg yolks, chilli, garlic, peanut butter and lemon juice in the bowl of a food processor and blend until creamy. With the motor running, gradually add the oil in a thin stream until the mixture thickens. Scrape out into a bowl and season to taste.

4 Lightly mix the minced beef with the breadcrumbs and season with salt and pepper. Shape into 4 patties, 2–3cm (¾–1¼ inches) thick.

5 Preheat a grill or griddle pan to medium–high and cook the patties for 4–5 minutes per side for rare to medium, or 8–10 minutes for medium to well done.

6 Lay the bases of the toasted buns on 4 serving plates, top with tomatoes, lettuce and the patties. Add a spoonful each of the peanut butter mayonnaise and bacon jam, top with the bun lids and serve.

LAURA PALMER'S TURKEY MELT BURGER

SERVES 4
PREPARATION TIME: 40 MINUTES
COOKING TIME: 20–25 MINUTES, PLUS
EXTRA FOR THE CREAMED CORN

25g (2 tablespoons) butter

finely grated zest and juice of ½ lemon

1 tablespoon chopped sage

1 garlic clove, crushed

4 spring onions, finely sliced

100ml (scant ½ cup) milk

25g (½ cup) day-old bread, broken into small pieces

500g (generous 2 cups) minced turkey

4 slices of smoked pancetta or streaky bacon

1 tablespoon olive oil

4 slices of Gruyère or other hard cheese

4 soft burger buns, split and toasted

salt and pepper

1 quantity of Garmonbozia Creamed Corn (*see* page 158), to serve

❶ Place the butter in a small saucepan over a medium heat, add the lemon zest, cook for 1 minute, then add the sage and garlic. Add the spring onions, cook for 2–3 minutes until softened, then pour in the milk.

❷ Remove from the heat, stir in the bread pieces and set aside to cool completely. Transfer the bread to a sieve and squeeze gently to remove the milk.

❸ Place the minced turkey in a large mixing bowl, add the squeezed bread and lemon juice and season well. Wet your hands a little and form the mixture into 4 patties, about 2cm (¾ inch) thick. Cut the pancetta or bacon slices in half and stretch a piece over each side of each burger, securing with cocktail sticks if necessary.

❹ Brush the burgers with the olive oil. Preheat a grill, griddle pan or barbecue to high and cook for 20–25 minutes or until cooked through, turning frequently. Lay a slice of Gruyère on the top of each burger and cook until melted. Place the burgers in the toasted buns and serve with the garmonbozia creamed corn.

The house used for the exterior shots of Laura Palmer's home changed between the pilot episode and the prequel film *Twin Peaks: Fire Walk With Me*. The house used in the pilot was in the town of Monroe, north of Fall City, but the one used in the film was in Everett, north of Seattle. The interior of the Everett house was used as the Palmer house in both.

BOBBY BRIGGS'S BBQ SPECIAL BURGER

SERVES 4
PREPARATION TIME: 30 MINUTES
COOKING TIME: 45 MINUTES

2kg (8½ cups) coarsely minced beef

75g (1½ cups) fresh breadcrumbs

6 spring onions, finely chopped

salt and pepper

BBQ sauce

200g (generous ¾ cup) tomato ketchup

150g (¾ cup) dark brown sugar

100ml (scant ½ cup) apple juice

100ml (scant ½ cup) bourbon whiskey

4 tablespoons apple cider vinegar

1 tablespoon Sriracha hot chilli sauce

1 tablespoon Dijon mustard

Mayonnaise and slaw

2 egg yolks

2 teaspoons Dijon mustard

1–2 tablespoons lemon juice

200ml (scant 1 cup) sunflower, groundnut, olive oil or a mixture

6 spring onions, chopped

½ white cabbage, finely shredded

4 carrots, cut into matchsticks

1 large beetroot, cut into matchsticks

To serve

8 slices of Swiss cheese

6 burger buns or brioche buns, split and toasted

soft lettuce leaves

tomato slices

8 streaky bacon rashers, dry-fried until crisp

❶ For the BBQ sauce, place all the ingredients in a heavy-based saucepan, bring to the boil, reduce the heat and simmer for 10–15 minutes or until the sauce is thickened. Allow to cool completely.

❷ Lightly mix the minced beef with the breadcrumbs and spring onions and season with salt and pepper. Shape into 8 patties, about 2cm (¾ inch) thick.

❸ For the mayonnaise, place the egg yolks, mustard and 1 tablespoon of lemon juice in a food processor and blend until thickened slightly. With the motor running, gradually add the oil in a thin, steady stream until the mixture thickens. Season and add more lemon juice, to taste.

❹ For the slaw, place the spring onions, cabbage, carrots and beetroot in a large mixing bowl with half the mayonnaise and mix thoroughly. Season to taste.

❺ Preheat a grill or griddle pan to medium–high and cook the patties for 4–5 minutes per side for rare to medium, or 8–10 minutes for medium to well done. Lay a slice of Swiss cheese on top of each burger during the last minute of cooking to soften.

❻ Lay a base of a toasted bun on a plate, top with lettuce, a spoonful of slaw, a burger, a couple of slices of tomato and a spoonful of the BBQ sauce. Add another piece of bun, more lettuce, then top with a second burger and repeat with the tomato, the BBQ sauce and finally balance 2 slices of bacon on top, then finish with the top of the bun to serve.

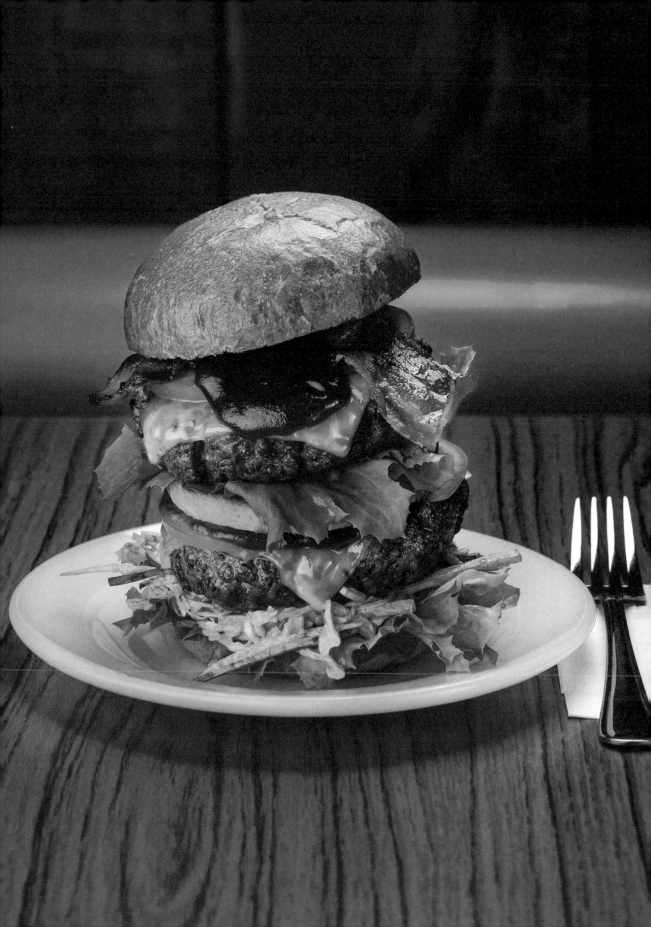

ICED TEA

SERVES 4
PREPARATION TIME: 10 MINUTES,
PLUS COOLING
COOKING TIME: 5 MINUTES

4 tea bags or 4 teaspoons leaf tea
1 litre (4¼ cups) boiling water
runny honey or sugar, to taste
ice cubes, to serve

❶ Place the tea bags or leaf tea into a heatproof jug and pour over the just-boiled water.

❷ Stir in honey or sugar to taste and leave to brew for about 5 minutes, then strain. Allow to cool, then place in the refrigerator to chill.

❸ To serve, pour the tea into glasses filled with ice cubes. Choose a garnish from the list below.

GARNISHES
- **English breakfast or Earl grey tea**: lemon slices
- **Ginger tea (add a few slices of fresh root ginger to the water when brewing)**: lemon, lime or orange slices
- **Green tea**: cucumber slices
- **Peppermint tea**: mint leaves
- **Summer berry tea**: fresh berries
- **Fruit teas**: mango or peach slices

CHOCOLATE & COFFEE SHAKE

SERVES 4
PREPARATION TIME: 15 MINUTES
COOKING TIME: 10 MINUTES

400ml (1⅔ cups) strong black espresso coffee

3 tablespoons dark soft brown sugar

100g (1 cup) plain dark chocolate (minimum 70% cocoa solids), broken into cubes

4 tablespoons malted milk drink powder (optional)

400ml (1⅔ cups) double cream

1½ teaspoons caster sugar

1 litre (4¼ cups) vanilla or coffee ice cream

Maltesers, to decorate (optional)

Chocolate sauce

100ml (scant ½ cup) double cream

75g (¾ cup) plain dark chocolate (minimum 70% cocoa solids), broken into cubes

❶ To make the milkshake base, heat the coffee in a pan, stir in the dark soft brown sugar, three-quarters of the chocolate and the malted milk drink powder (if using) and stir until melted. Remove from the heat, pour into a jug and allow to cool.

❷ For the chocolate sauce, place the cream in a small saucepan set over a low heat and bring slowly to the boil. Remove from the heat, add the chocolate and stir until melted and smooth. Scrape into a bowl and place in the refrigerator to cool but not set.

❸ Finely chop the remaining chocolate. Whip the cream with the caster sugar until soft peaks form, then stir in half of the chopped chocolate. Set aside.

❹ Once the milkshake base has cooled, pour one-quarter of the mixture into a blender, add one-quarter of the ice cream and blend until smooth. Pour into a tall glass, top with some of the whipped cream, drizzle with a little of the chocolate sauce and sprinkle with a little of the remaining chopped chocolate. Repeat with the remaining ingredients to make 4 shakes and serve immediately, decorated with Maltesers, if using.

See photograph, page 69.

COCONUT & LIME SHAKE

SERVES 1
PREPARATION TIME: 30 MINUTES
COOKING TIME: 25–30 MINUTES

2 mature coconuts, or 400ml (1⅔ cups) canned coconut milk

300ml (1¼ cups) warm water (optional)

2 teaspoons desiccated coconut

100ml (scant ½ cup) double cream

2 teaspoons caster sugar

finely grated zest of ½ lime

6 scoops (generous 1 cup) of ice cream

1 tablespoon maple syrup or honey

2 teaspoons lime juice

1 To make fresh coconut milk, preheat the oven to 180°C (350°F), Gas Mark 4. Pierce the 2 soft eyes in the coconut shells and drain out the coconut water. Bake the coconuts in the oven for 20–30 minutes until the shells crack open. Alternatively, break the shells with a hammer.

2 Take the flesh out of the coconuts and remove the hard brown skin. Place the flesh in a food processor with the measured warm water and blend until finely shredded. Tip the mixture into a sieve lined with muslin or a clean tea towel, set over a bowl. Gather up the cloth, squeeze out the milk and place in the refrigerator to chill. Alternatively, use canned coconut milk.

3 Place the desiccated coconut in a dry frying pan and toast over a medium heat, stirring occasionally, for about 5 minutes until just turning golden. Tip out on to a plate to cool completely.

4 Whip the cream with the sugar and lime zest until soft peaks form.

5 Pour 400ml (1⅔ cups) of the coconut milk into a blender with the ice cream, maple syrup and lime juice, and blend until smooth. Pour the shake into a tall glass, top with the whipped cream, sprinkle with the toasted coconut and serve immediately.

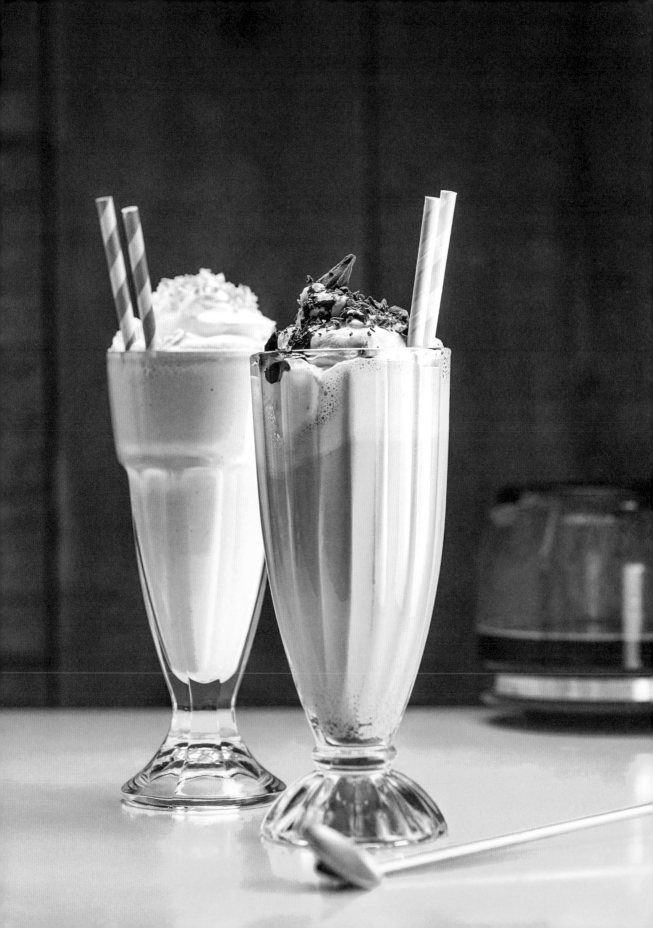

HOMEMADE CHERRY COLA

SERVES 4–6
PREPARATION TIME: 30 MINUTES,
PLUS OVERNIGHT MARINATING
COOKING TIME: 15 MINUTES

350g (1½ cups) cherries

2 vanilla pods

300g (1½ cups) golden caster sugar

75g (generous ½ cup) raw cocao nibs

1 tablespoon dried lavender flowers

3 x 10-cm (4-inch) cinnamon sticks

finely grated zest of 1 large lemon

finely grated zest of 1 large lime

finely grated zest of 2 oranges

300ml (1¼ cups) water

1 teaspoon citric acid

2 whole nutmegs or ¼ teaspoon
ground nutmeg

1 star anise

½ teaspoon ground ginger

To serve

ice cubes

1–1.5 litres (5 cups) soda water

❶ Remove the stones from the cherries and place the flesh in a large saucepan. Crack the cherry stones with a pair of pliers and place them in the pan. Split the vanilla pods lengthways with the tip of a sharp knife and remove the seeds by scraping the knife down the insides of the pods. Place the seeds and pods in the pan with the cherries.

❷ Add all the remaining ingredients and place over a medium heat, stirring until the sugar has dissolved. Bring to a simmer and cook gently for about 5 minutes until the cherries are tender. Remove from the heat, cover and leave overnight.

❸ When ready to use, tip the cherry mixture into a sieve set over a bowl and press the fruit with the back of a spoon to extract all the juice.

❹ To serve, half-fill a glass with ice and drizzle over 4 tablespoons of the cherry syrup. Top up with about 250ml (generous 1 cup) of soda water and stir well. Serve immediately.

HOMEMADE LEMONADE

SERVES 4–6
PREPARATION TIME: 10 MINUTES,
PLUS COOLING
COOKING TIME: 15 MINUTES

6 juicy unwaxed lemons

150g (¾ cup) golden caster sugar or 250g (generous 1 cup) runny honey

1 litre (4¼ cups) water

To serve

sparkling or still water, to dilute

ice cubes

❶ Finely grate the zest from 3 of the lemons and place in a large saucepan with the sugar or honey and the measured water. Bring to the boil, stirring to dissolve the sugar, then remove from the heat.

❷ Squeeze the juice from all the lemons. This should give you 200–250ml (scant 1 cup–generous 1 cup) of juice.

❸ Strain the lemon zest liquid through a sieve into a jug and stir in lemon juice to taste. Stir well and leave to cool, then chill in the refrigerator.

❹ To serve, dilute the lemonade with sparkling or still water, to taste, and add ice cubes. Serve immediately.

CORN DOGS

MAKES 20
PREPARATION TIME: 20 MINUTES
**COOKING TIME: 15 MINUTES, PLUS EXTRA
FOR THE CREAMED CORN, IF MAKING**

100g (⅔ cup) yellow cornmeal or polenta

100g (generous ¾ cup) plain flour

1 teaspoon sea salt

½ teaspoon ground black pepper

1 teaspoon baking powder

¼ teaspoon bicarbonate of soda

¼ teaspoon cayenne pepper

200g (scant 1 cup) canned cream-style corn, or Garmonbozia Creamed Corn (see page 158)

½ small onion, grated

1 jalapeño or other green chilli, deseeded and finely chopped

200ml (scant 1 cup) buttermilk, or 1 egg mixed with 150ml (⅔ cup) milk

10 hot dogs

groundnut oil, for deep-frying

mustard and ketchup, to serve

❶ Place the cornmeal, flour, salt, pepper, baking powder, bicarbonate of soda and cayenne pepper in a mixing bowl and mix well.

❷ Place the creamed corn, onion, chilli and buttermilk (or egg and milk) in another bowl and beat together. Cut the hot dogs in half and skewer each half lengthways on a wooden skewer.

❸ Heat the oil in a large, deep saucepan or deep-fat fryer to 180–190°C (350–375°F) or until a cube of bread browns in 30 seconds.

❹ Pour the wet ingredients into the bowl with the dry ingredients and mix well. Pour some of the mixture into a tall glass. Dip the skewered hot dogs, one at a time, into the batter to coat evenly. Lift them out, shaking off any excess batter, then lower carefully into the hot oil. Cook in batches to avoid crowding the pan.

❺ Fry the corn dogs for 1–2 minutes on each side, turning occasionally, or until golden and puffy on all sides. Drain on kitchen paper, then cool for 5 minutes before serving with mustard and ketchup.

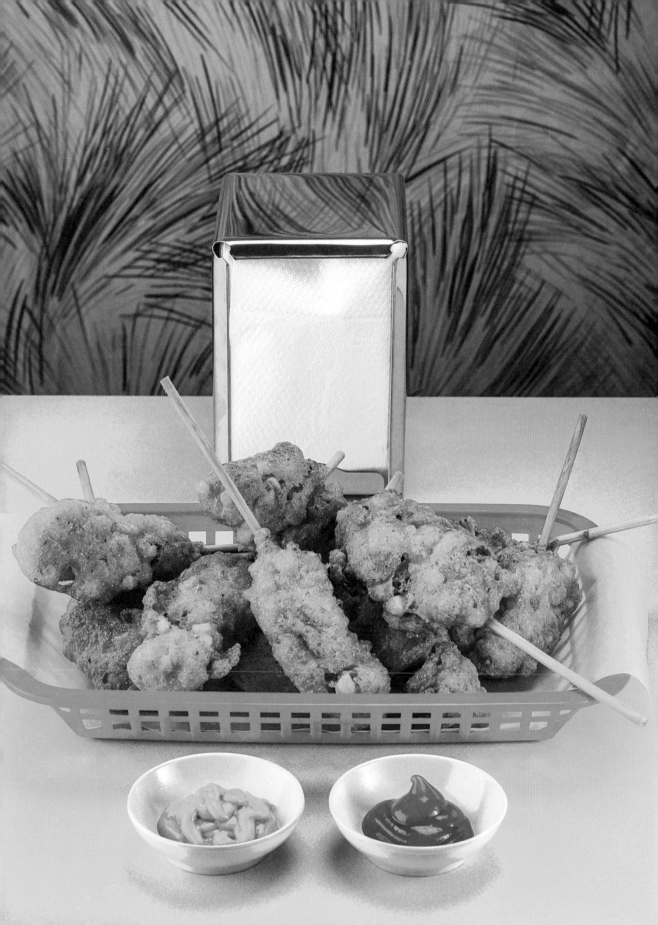

HAWAIIAN PINEAPPLE RELISH

SERVES 4–6 AS A SIDE
PREPARATION TIME: 15 MINUTES

1 small pineapple, peeled, cored and finely chopped

½ small red onion, finely chopped

3 tablespoons lime juice

finely grated zest of 1 lime

2.5-cm (1-inch) piece of fresh root ginger, peeled and finely grated

1 garlic clove, crushed

1 teaspoon apple cider vinegar

½ teaspoon Chinese five-spice powder

1 red chilli, deseeded and finely chopped

salt and pepper

1 tablespoon chopped toasted peanuts, to garnish

❶ Place all the ingredients, except the peanuts and seasoning, in a large mixing bowl and toss together well.

❷ Just before serving, season to taste and arrange in a serving dish. If you add salt too early, it will draw moisture out of the ingredients, making the relish wet. Scatter over the peanuts and serve immediately.

ANNIE BLACKBURN'S CORN BREAD

SERVES 6–8 AS A SIDE
PREPARATION TIME: 20 MINUTES
COOKING TIME: 40–50 MINUTES

200g (1⅓ cups) coarse yellow cornmeal, preferably stoneground

2 sweetcorn cobs, husks and silks removed

75g (5 tablespoons) butter

200g (scant 1⅔ cups) plain flour

½ teaspoon salt

2 teaspoons baking powder

¼ teaspoon bicarbonate of soda

1–3 tablespoons light soft brown sugar, to taste

300ml (1¼ cups) buttermilk or milk

3 eggs, beaten

50g (½ cup) Parmesan cheese, finely grated (optional)

pepper

❶ Place the cornmeal in a dry frying pan over a medium heat and toast, stirring frequently, until it starts to smell fragrant. Remove from the heat and set aside.

❷ Use a large, sharp knife to trim the tops and bottoms from the sweetcorn cobs. One at a time, stand them on their bases and cut the kernels off the cobs from top to bottom, turning as you go. Then, with the point of a spoon, scrape down the cobs to remove any pulp.

❸ Preheat the oven to 220°C (425°F), Gas Mark 7. Melt the butter in a 24-cm (9½-inch) ovenproof frying pan over a medium heat until it is just starting to brown, taking care not to burn it. Add the corn kernels, season well with black pepper, reduce the heat and cook for 5–10 minutes until tender.

❹ Place the remaining ingredients, including the cornmeal, in a large bowl and mix to create a smooth batter. Turn up the heat under the frying pan and pour in the batter; it should sizzle as it hits the pan. Transfer the pan to the oven and cook for about 35–40 minutes until golden brown and firm in the middle. Serve warm, cut into cubes.

CHILLI-BRUSHED CORN

SERVES 4
PREPARATION TIME: 15 MINUTES
COOKING TIME: 4–5 MINUTES

200g (1¾ sticks) butter, softened

6 tablespoons finely chopped dill

2 red chillies, deseeded and finely chopped

4 sweetcorn cobs, husk and silks removed

1 Place the butter, dill and chilli in a bowl and beat until smooth. Set aside.

2 Cut each sweetcorn cob into 3 equal-sized pieces. Insert a wooden or metal skewer into the side of each piece. Preheat a barbecue or griddle pan to high and cook, turning frequently, for 4–5 minutes or until lightly charred and blistered in places.

3 Brush the corn with the butter and serve immediately.

GARLIC BREAD

SERVES 2
PREPARATION TIME: 5 MINUTES
COOKING TIME: 4 MINUTES

4 slices of bread, such as ciabatta, sourdough, baguette or pitta

2–3 garlic cloves, peeled and halved

8 tablespoons olive oil

chopped flat leaf parsley, to sprinkle (optional)

salt

1 Preheat a grill to medium and toast the bread on both sides until golden. While the bread is still warm, rub one side with the cut sides of the garlic.

2 Put the warm toasted bread on a plate and drizzle 2 tablespoons of the olive oil over each slice. Sprinkle with salt and a little chopped parsley, if liked, and serve as a starter or side.

GARLIC FRIES

SERVES 4
PREPARATION TIME: 20 MINUTES
COOKING TIME: 20 MINUTES

1kg (2lb 4 oz) floury potatoes

2 litres (8½ cups) groundnut, corn
or sunflower oil for deep-frying or
4 tablespoons oil for oven baking

100g (7 tablespoons) butter

4 garlic cloves, crushed

2 tablespoons chopped flat leaf parsley

salt and pepper

1 Cut the potatoes into 5-mm (¼-inch) slices, leaving the skin on. Cut the slices into 5-mm (¼-inch) fries, rinse thoroughly in cold water to remove surface starch and drain well. Pat the fries with a clean tea towel, transfer to another clean dry tea towel and dry again.

2 To deep-fry, pour the oil into a large, deep saucepan or deep-fat fryer, making sure it is no more than one-third to one-half full. Heat the oil until it reaches 160°C (325°F). Carefully lower the fries, in batches, into the hot oil and cook for 5 minutes until tender but still pale. Drain well on kitchen paper.

3 Meanwhile, place the butter and garlic in a small saucepan over a medium–low heat. Cook for 2–3 minutes until the garlic is softened but not coloured. Remove from the heat, season with lots of pepper and stir in the chopped parsley.

4 Raise the heat of the oil to 190°C (375°F) and carefully lower the blanched fries back into the oil, again in batches. Cook for 1–2 minutes until golden brown and crisp. Drain well on kitchen paper.

5 Alternatively, to oven bake the fries, preheat the oven to 220°C (425°F), Gas Mark 7. Place the fries with 4 tablespoons of oil in a large bowl and toss to coat, then arrange them in a single layer on 2 baking sheets. Cook for about 30 minutes, shaking the trays and turning the fries occasionally, until golden and crispy. Drain well on kitchen paper.

6 Tip the fries into a bowl, pour over the garlic butter, season with salt and toss well to coat. Serve immediately.

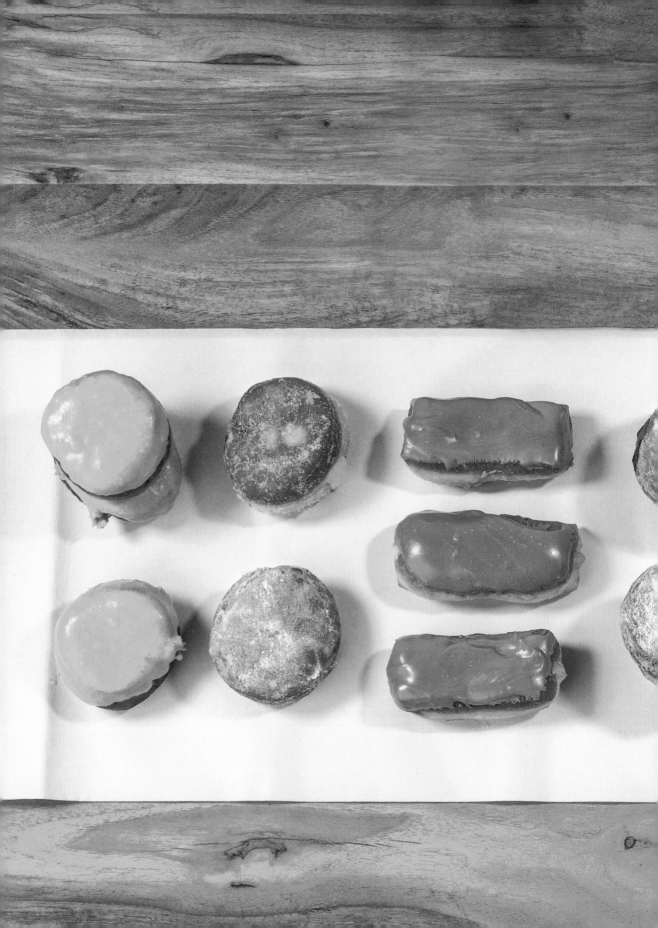

chapter 3

DONUTS & PASTRIES

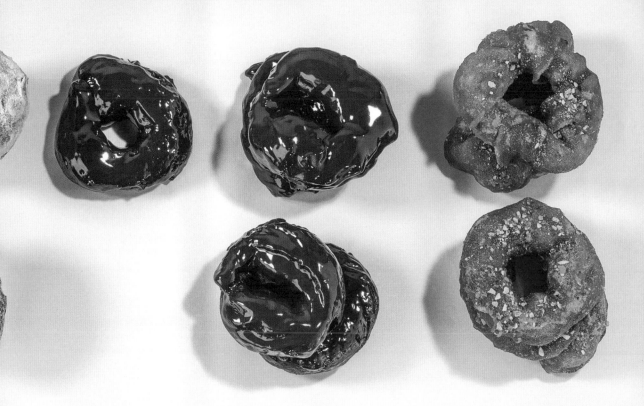

DONUTS & PASTRIES

Donuts, donuts, donuts! *Twin Peaks* seems to be full of them. And why not? They are, after all, a staple item in the local Sheriff Department's diet. Agent Cooper's favourite is the jelly donut, laid out by Lucy lovingly every night in the conference room. In fact, have you noticed that a donut doesn't appear in *Twin Peaks* unless it's connected to the Sheriff and his team in some way?

In this chapter we're taking the donuts out of the Sheriff's Department and into your kitchen! You'll find some recipes here that will have you salivating faster than Deputy Brennan can unravel sticky tape (okay, maybe that's not that fast…) and there are plenty of other pastries here to hit that spot too. It's a law enforcer's dream!

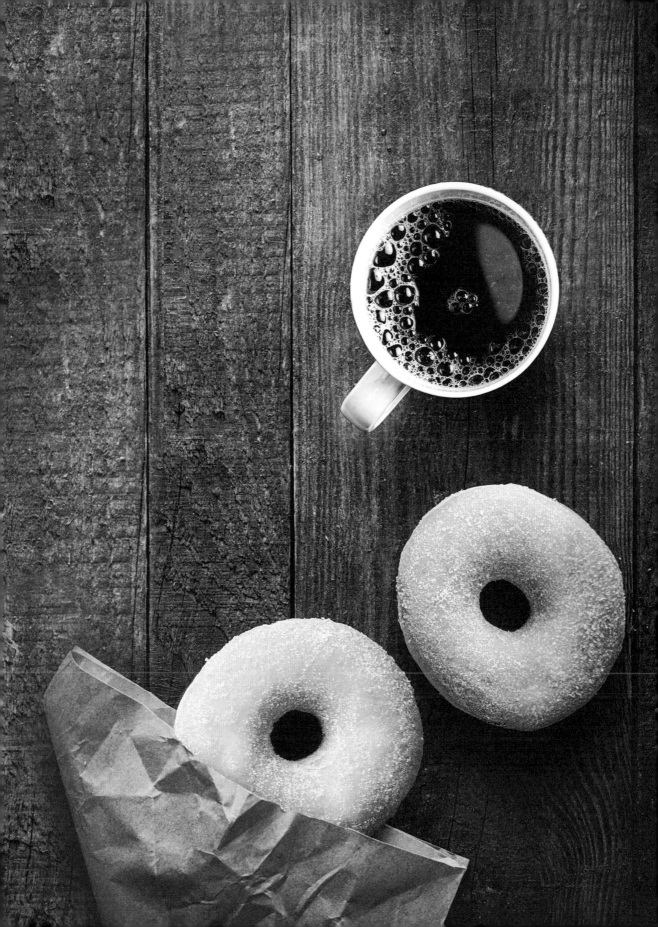

CINNAMON BEAR CLAWS

MAKES 10
**PREPARATION TIME: 45 MINUTES,
PLUS RISING**
COOKING TIME: 15–20 MINUTES

500g (3¾ cups) strong white flour

50g (¼ cup) caster sugar

1½ teaspoons salt

1½ teaspoons fast-action dried yeast or
15g (½oz) fresh yeast, crumbled

4 eggs

finely grated zest of 1 lemon

200ml (scant 1 cup) milk or water, warmed

200g (1¾ sticks) unsalted butter, cubed,
at room temperature

Filling and topping
250g (9oz) marzipan

1 large egg, separated

50g (scant ¼ cup) caster sugar

1 teaspoon ground cinnamon

50g (½ cup) almonds, finely sliced

Glaze
100g (generous ¼ cup) runny honey

2 tablespoons milk

1 teaspoon vanilla extract

❶ Place the flour, sugar, salt, yeast, eggs, lemon zest and milk or water into a mixer fitted with a dough hook and mix for 6–8 minutes or until the dough forms a ball. Gradually add the butter in small pieces until incorporated, then continue to mix for about 5 minutes or until the dough is glossy and elastic. Alternatively, mix the ingredients by hand in a mixing bowl and knead on a lightly floured surface.

❷ Cover the bowl with clingfilm and leave in a warm place for 1–1½ hours until doubled in size.

❸ Tip the dough out on to a lightly floured surface and knead to knock out all the air, then place back in the bowl, cover and refrigerate for at least 6 hours or overnight.

❹ For the filling, place the marzipan in a bowl and gradually knead in the egg white, sugar and cinnamon until well incorporated. Set aside.

❺ Preheat the oven to 200°C (400°F), Gas Mark 6 and line 2 baking sheets with baking parchment. Knead the dough briefly to knock all the air out of it, then cut in half. Roll each piece out on a lightly floured surface to form a 40 x 20-cm (16 x 8-inch) rectangle. Divide the almond mixture between the rectangles and spread evenly over the surface using a spoon or a knife and leaving a 1-cm (½-inch) gap all around.

❻ Gently roll up the rectangles from their longest edges to form 2 long sausages. Brush all over with the egg yolk and cut each into 5 equal pieces. Use a small knife or scissors to make 5 cuts along one edge of each pastry, from the edge to the middle.

❼ Arrange the pastries on the lined baking sheets, slightly opening the gaps as you go. Sprinkle with the sliced almonds and cook for 15–20 minutes or until golden. Cool on a wire rack.

❽ For the glaze, place the honey, milk and vanilla in a small saucepan over a medium heat and bring to the boil. Drizzle the glaze over the pastries and leave to cool completely.

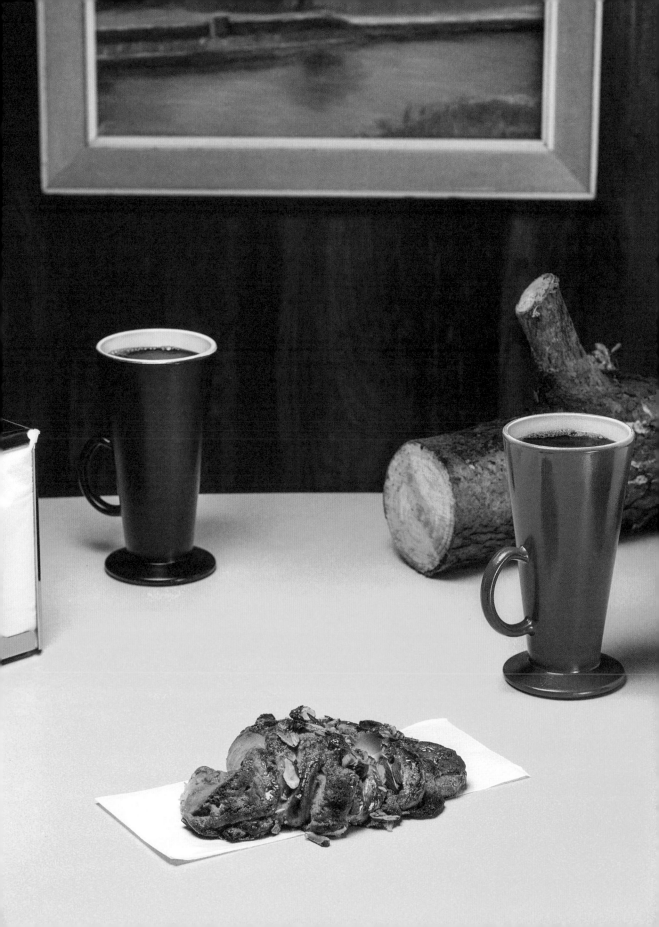

APPLE BUTTERSCOTCH TURNOVERS

MAKES 6
**PREPARATION TIME: 20 MINUTES,
PLUS COOLING AND CHILLING
COOKING TIME: 30–40 MINUTES**

25g (2 tablespoons) unsalted butter

3 tablespoons light soft brown sugar

1 tablespoon lemon juice

4 eating apples, peeled, cored and chopped

¼ teaspoon ground cinnamon

2 tablespoons sultanas

100ml (scant ½ cup) double cream

375g (13oz) puff pastry

1 egg, beaten

2 tablespoons demerara sugar

❶ Melt the butter and light soft brown sugar in a saucepan over a medium heat, add the lemon juice, apples and cinnamon and cook for about 5 minutes until the sugar starts to caramelize. Stir in the sultanas and cream and cook gently for a further 5–10 minutes or until the apples are tender and the mixture has thickened. Set aside to cool completely.

❷ Roll out the pastry on a lightly floured surface into a 5-mm (¼-inch) thick rectangle. Trim the edges with a sharp knife, then cut into 6 squares.

❸ Spoon the apple mixture into the centres of the pastry squares, brush the edges with a little beaten egg and fold over the pastry and tuck in the edges to form triangles. Use a fork to press the edges of the turnovers to seal.

❹ Arrange the turnovers on a baking sheet lined with baking parchment and chill in the refrigerator for 20 minutes. Preheat the oven to 200°C (400°F), Gas Mark 6.

❺ Brush the pastries all over with the remaining beaten egg, sprinkle with demerara sugar and make a small hole in the top of each to allow steam to escape. Bake for about 20 minutes or until golden and crisp. Allow to cool for 15 minutes before serving.

CINNAMON SUGAR PRETZELS

MAKES 16
PREPARATION TIME: 40 MINUTES
COOKING TIME: 40 MINUTES

2½ teaspoons fast-action dried yeast or 30g (1oz) fresh yeast, crumbled

1 teaspoon salt

2 tablespoons caster sugar

550g (4 cups) strong white flour

350ml (1½ cups) milk

100g (7 tablespoons) butter

600ml (2½ cups) water

2 tablespoons bicarbonate of soda

Coating

75g (5 tablespoons) butter, melted

2 teaspoons ground cinnamon

75g (generous ⅓ cup) caster sugar

❶ Place the yeast, salt, sugar and flour in a large bowl. Place the milk and butter in a saucepan and heat gently until the butter melts.

❷ Gradually pour the milk and butter mixture into the bowl with the flour and combine with a fork, then your hands, to form a soft dough. Knead the dough on a lightly floured surface for 8–10 minutes until shiny and elastic.

❸ Cut the dough into 16 equal pieces. To shape the pretzels, roll each piece into a sausage about 60cm (24 inches) long and arrange into a U-shape on the work surface. Twist the two sides over each other twice, then bring the ends towards you and press one on each side of the bottom of the U to attach. Arrange the pretzels on 2 baking sheets lined with baking parchment.

❹ Bring the measured water to the boil in a large saucepan, remove from the heat and add the bicarbonate of soda. Place back on the heat and lower a pretzel into the water. Simmer for 2 minutes on one side, then turn over and cook for 1 minute more. Carefully lift out, shaking off any excess water, and return to the baking sheet. Repeat with the remaining pretzels.

❺ Preheat the oven to 200°C (400°F), Gas Mark 6 and cook the pretzels for 8–10 minutes until rich golden brown.

❻ Meanwhile, make the coating by placing all the ingredients in a small saucepan over a gentle heat and stirring until the sugar has dissolved. Remove the pretzels from the oven and brush with the butter mixture while still warm.

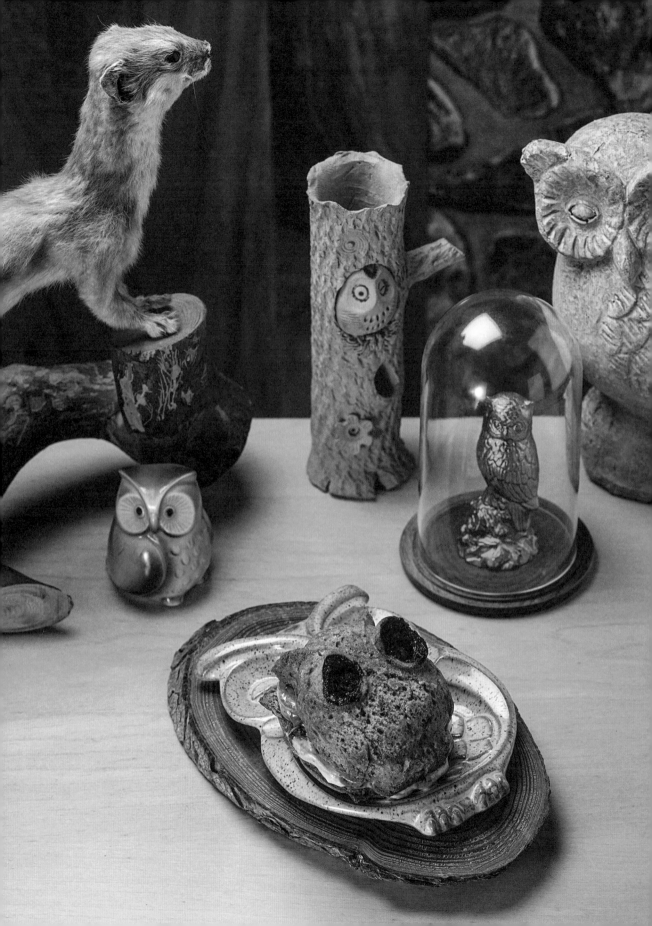

BLUEBERRY WHOOPIE PIES

MAKES 15
PREPARATION TIME: 30 MINUTES
COOKING TIME: 15–20 MINUTES

100g (7 tablespoons) butter, softened

200g (1 cup) caster sugar

½ teaspoon vanilla extract

1 large egg, beaten

50ml (scant ¼ cup) buttermilk

325g (2⅔ cups) plain flour

½ teaspoon baking powder

½ teaspoon salt

30 blueberries

Blueberry purée

200g (2 cups) blueberries

2 tablespoons caster sugar

1 teaspoon vanilla extract

2 teaspoons water

Filling

300g (1⅓ cups) cream cheese or mascarpone

50g (½ cup) icing sugar, plus extra for dusting

pinch of salt

½ teaspoon vanilla extract

① For the blueberry purée, place all the ingredients in a small saucepan over a medium heat. Bring to the boil and boil rapidly for 2–3 minutes. Crush the berries with the back of a spoon, then reduce the heat and simmer for 5–8 minutes or until very tender and thickened. Leave to cool completely.

② Preheat the oven to 170°C (338°F), Gas Mark 3½ and line 2 baking sheets with baking parchment.

③ Place the butter, sugar and vanilla extract in a large mixing bowl and beat until smooth. Place the egg, buttermilk and half the cooled blueberry purée in a jug and beat to combine, then beat the mixture into the butter and sugar mixture. Sieve the flour, baking powder and salt into a bowl, then fold the dry ingredients into the wet ingredients.

④ Spoon 30 mounds of batter, each about 5cm (2 inches) across, on to the lined baking sheets, leaving space for them to spread. Top each mound with a whole blueberry and cook in the oven for 10–15 minutes or until the sponge bounces back when lightly touched. Allow to cool completely.

⑤ For the filling, beat the cream cheese with the icing sugar, salt, vanilla and the remaining blueberry purée until smooth and creamy. Use the filling to sandwich the cooled whoopie pies together in pairs.

VARIATION: BLUEBERRY WHOOPIE OWLS

Use silicon owl moulds to create 12 Blueberry Whoopie Owls (using the extra blueberries for googly eyes – see photograph) from the ingredients above. Once the pies are baked, carefully cut the owls in half and sandwich with filling as with the Whoopie Pies.

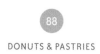
RASPBERRY GARLANDS

MAKES 8
PREPARATION TIME: 30 MINUTES
COOKING TIME: 15 MINUTES

150ml (⅔ cup) water

50g (3½ tablespoons) butter, plus extra
for greasing

65g (½ cup) plain flour, sifted

2 eggs, beaten

½ teaspoon vanilla essence

15g (scant ¼ cup) flaked almonds

sifted icing sugar, for dusting

Filling

300ml (1¼ cups) full-fat crème fraîche

3 tablespoons icing sugar, sifted

250g (2 cups) fresh raspberries

1 Heat the measured water and butter gently in a saucepan until melted. Bring to the boil, then add the flour and beat until it forms a smooth ball that leaves the sides of the pan almost clean. Allow to cool for 10 minutes.

2 Preheat the oven to 200°C (400°F), Gas Mark 6. Gradually mix in the eggs and vanilla until thick and smooth. Spoon the choux mixture into a large nylon piping bag fitted with a 1-cm (½-inch) plain piping tube and pipe 7.5-cm (3-inch) diameter circles on a greased baking sheet.

3 Sprinkle with the flaked almonds, then bake in the oven for 15 minutes. Make a small slit in the side of each choux ring for the steam to escape, then return to the turned-off oven for 5 minutes. Leave to cool.

4 Slit each choux ring and fill with crème fraîche mixed with half the icing sugar, then sprinkle with the raspberries. Arrange on a serving plate and dust with the remaining icing sugar. These are best eaten on the day they are made.

CHOCOLATE ÉCLAIRS WITH CREAM LIQUEUR

MAKES 18
PREPARATION TIME: 40 MINUTES,
COOKING TIME: 15 MINUTES
PLUS COOLING

150ml (⅔ cup) water

50g (3½ tablespoons) butter, plus extra
for greasing

65g (½ cup) plain flour, sifted

2 eggs, beaten

½ teaspoon vanilla essence

Filling

240ml (1 cup) double cream

2 tablespoons icing sugar

4 tablespoons cream liqueur
(such as Baileys)

Topping

25g (2 tablespoons) butter

100g (scant ⅔ cup) plain dark
chocolate (minimum 70% cocoa solids),
chopped

1 tablespoon icing sugar

2–3 teaspoons milk

❶ Place the measured water and butter in a saucepan over a medium heat and bring to the boil. Add the flour and beat vigorously until the mixture forms a smooth ball that leaves the sides of the pan. Leave to cool for 10 minutes. Preheat the oven to 200°C (400°F), Gas Mark 6.

❷ Gradually beat in the eggs and vanilla essence until thick and smooth. Spoon the choux mixture into a large nylon piping bag fitted with a 1-cm (½-inch) plain nozzle and pipe 7.5-cm (3-inch) lines of mixture on to a large lightly greased baking sheet. Bake for 15 minutes until well risen, then turn off the oven.

❸ Make a slit in the side of each éclair for the steam to escape, then return to the oven for 5 minutes. Leave to cool.

❹ For the filling, whip the cream until soft peaks form, then gradually stir in the icing sugar and liqueur. Slit each éclair lengthways and spoon or pipe in the filling.

❺ For the topping, place the butter, chocolate and icing sugar in a saucepan over a gentle heat until just melted. Stir in the milk, then spoon over the tops of the éclairs. Serve the same day.

THE BIG DONUT QUIZ

Every Twin Peaks fan knows that donuts are key to the show and appear in nearly every episode! Have this quiz to hand next time you are watching Twin Peaks, or test your friends at a dinner party inspired by Twin Peaks. Can you spot the donut references and answer the questions below?

1 How many donuts (to the nearest billion) are produced in the US each year?

2 In the pilot of *Twin Peaks*, what does Lucy say there is extra of for Agent Cooper?

3 In the Season 2 opener, what does Agent Cooper answer when Sheriff Truman asks him if he wants coffee and donuts for when he "lays the whole thing out"?

4 How many people in the US (to the nearest 10) have the surname Donut or Doughnut?

5 How many donuts a day did Renée Zellweger say she ate to gain weight to play Bridget Jones?

6 Where is Agent Cooper when he says the line "Gimme a donut"?

7 Where does Lucy keep the donuts at the Sheriff's Station before she distributes them in the conference room, and in what colour boxes are they stored?

8 Just before Judge Sternwood enters the Sheriff's Station, Lucy is standing drinking, staring at donuts. Which famous face is on the mug next to the donuts?

9 Just before the One-Armed Man (Philip Gerard AKA Mike) is taken to the Great Northern Hotel to see if he can find BOB, there are five people with him in the Sheriff's Station standing in a line drinking coffee and eating donuts – can you name them all?

10 When Agent Cooper is sitting in the conference room going through the torn-up pieces of Laura Palmer's secret diary, how many donuts are on the plate in front of him?

11 When Sheriff Truman walks into his office eating a jelly donut and sees Catherine Martell leaning against his desk, what is the first thing he says to her?

12 What is behind the table full of donuts in the Tibetan Rock Throwing scene?

13 In what year was the first donut machine made?

14 What does Agent Cooper first say when he sees the donuts Lucy has laid out in the pilot?

15 Which US city has the most donut shops per person?

SHERIFF TRUMAN'S SUGAR-COATED RING DONUTS

MAKES 20
PREPARATION TIME: 45 MINUTES,
PLUS RISING AND CHILLING
COOKING TIME: ABOUT 25 MINUTES

500g (scant 3¾ cups) strong white flour

50g (¼ cup) caster sugar, plus extra
for coating

1½ teaspoons salt

1½ teaspoons fast-action dried yeast or
15g (½oz) fresh yeast, crumbled

4 eggs

finely grated zest of 1 lemon

200ml (scant 1 cup) milk or water, warmed

125g (1⅛ sticks) unsalted butter, cubed,
at room temperature

groundnut oil, for deep-frying

❶ Place the flour, sugar, salt, yeast, eggs, lemon zest and milk or water into a mixer fitted with a dough hook and mix for 6–8 minutes or until the dough forms a ball. Gradually add the butter in small pieces until incorporated, then continue to mix for about 5 minutes or until the dough is glossy and elastic. Alternatively, mix the ingredients by hand in a mixing bowl and knead on a lightly floured surface.

❷ Cover the bowl with clingfilm and leave in a warm place for 1–1½ hours until doubled in size.

❸ Tip the dough out on to a floured surface and knead to knock out all the air, then place back in the bowl, cover and refrigerate for at least 6 hours or overnight.

❹ Roll out the dough on a lightly floured surface to about 1cm (½ inch) thick. Use an 8-cm (3¼-inch) cutter to cut out rounds, then cut a hole out of the middle of each using a 3-cm (1¼-inch) cutter. Arrange the donuts on a lightly greased tray, leaving space for them to expand. Lightly cover with greased clingfilm and leave in a warm place for about 4 hours or until doubled in size.

❺ To deep-fry, pour the oil into a large, deep saucepan or deep-fat fryer, making sure it is no more than one-third to one-half full. Heat the oil until it reaches 180°C (350°F) or until a cube of bread browns in 30 seconds.

❻ Carefully lower about 3 donuts at a time into the hot oil and fry for 2–3 minutes on each side until golden brown. Remove with a slotted spoon and drain on kitchen paper. When cool enough to handle, toss them, one at a time, in caster sugar to coat and serve warm or cold.

CHERRY DONUTS

MAKES 20
PREPARATION TIME: 45 MINUTES,
PLUS RISING AND CHILLING
COOKING TIME: ABOUT 1 HOUR

1 quantity donut dough (see page 91)

groundnut oil, for deep-frying

caster sugar, for coating

Cherry filling

550g (2½ cups) sweet cherries, pitted and chopped

2 tablespoons water

juice of 2 lemons

350g (1⅔ cups) jam sugar with pectin

❶ For the filling, place the cherries and any juice with the measured water in a saucepan over a medium heat. Bring to the boil, reduce the heat and simmer for 15–20 minutes until tender.

❷ Add the lemon juice and sugar, stir until dissolved, then increase the heat and boil for 10–15 minutes, stirring occasionally. To test the set, place a teaspoonful of the mixture on a saucer and place in the freezer until cool. If your finger leaves a clear trail when you drag it through the mixture, the filling is ready. Allow to cool until just warm then purée in a blender until smooth (this makes it easier to pipe into the donuts).

❸ Make the dough and cook the donuts following the instructions on page 91, rolling the dough into 20 balls about the size of a golf ball rather than cutting it into rings. Toss the cooked donuts in caster sugar as soon as they are fried and drained, then leave to cool for 30 minutes.

❹ Fit a piping bag with a plain nozzle large enough for the filling to pass through. Spoon the filling into the bag, insert the nozzle into the side of a cooked donut and squeeze until it plumps up slightly. Repeat with the remaining donuts.

VARIATION: BLUEBERRY FILLING

350g (3½ cups) blueberries

1 tablespoon water

finely grated zest and juice of 2 lemons

300g (1½ cups) jam sugar with pectin

❶ Place the blueberries and measured water in a saucepan over a medium heat. Bring to the boil, reduce the heat and simmer for 5 minutes until tender.

❷ Add the lemon zest, juice and sugar, stir until dissolved, then increase the heat and boil for 10–15 minutes, stirring occasionally. To test the set, place a teaspoonful of the mixture on a saucer and place in the freezer until cool. If your finger leaves a clear trail when you drag it through the mixture, the filling is ready. Allow to cool until just warm then purée in a blender until smooth.

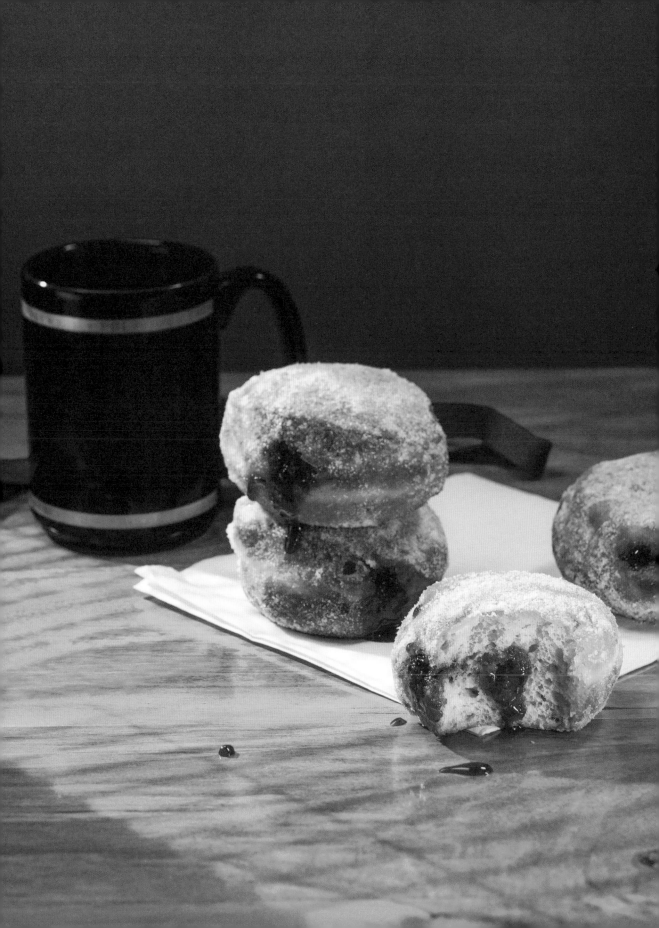

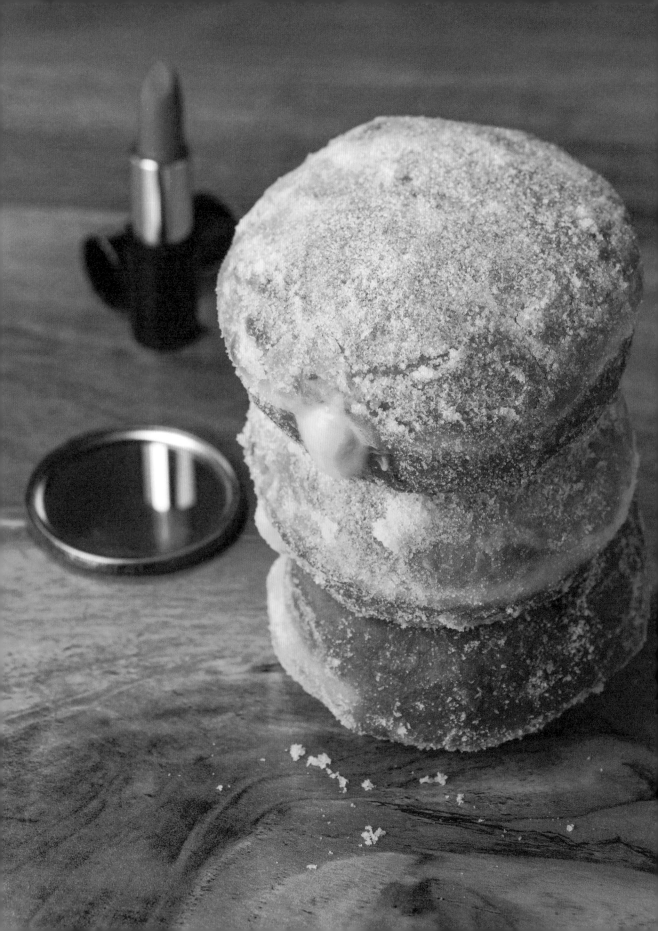

DENISE BRYSON'S LEMON & WHITE CHOCOLATE DONUTS

MAKES 20
PREPARATION TIME: 1 HOUR 15 MINUTES, PLUS RISING AND CHILLING
COOKING TIME: ABOUT 1 HOUR

200ml (scant 1 cup) double cream

1 tablespoon caster sugar

4 tablespoons lemon curd

1 quantity donut dough (see page 91)

groundnut oil, for deep-frying

caster sugar, for coating

Custard base

6 egg yolks

150g (¾ cup) caster sugar, plus
2 tablespoons

75g (generous ½ cup) plain flour

500ml (generous 2 cups) milk

1 vanilla pod, split lengthways

200g (generous 1 cup) white chocolate,
finely chopped

❶ For the custard, place the egg yolks and sugar in a mixing bowl and whisk for 2 minutes until pale, then whisk in the flour thoroughly.

❷ Place the milk and vanilla pod in a small saucepan over a medium heat and bring to the boil. Pour the boiling milk over the egg yolk mixture and whisk until well combined.

❸ Pour the mixture back into the pan over a low heat and bring back to the boil, whisking all the time until very thick and smooth. Remove from the heat and beat in the white chocolate until melted. Cover the surface with clingfilm to prevent a skin forming and leave to cool.

❹ Whip the cream with the remaining 2 tablespoons caster sugar until soft peaks form, then fold into the cooled custard. Finally, marble the lemon curd through the mixture and refrigerate until needed.

❺ Make the dough and cook the donuts following the instructions on page 91, rolling the dough into 20 balls about the size of a golf ball rather than cutting it into rings. Toss the cooked donuts in caster sugar as soon as they are fried and drained, then leave to cool for 30 minutes.

❻ Fit a piping bag with a plain nozzle large enough for the filling to pass through. Spoon the filling into the bag, insert the nozzle into the side of a cooked donut and squeeze until it plumps up slightly. Repeat with the remaining donuts.

LUCY MORAN'S COFFEE DONUTS

MAKES 20
PREPARATION TIME: 1 HOUR 15 MINUTES,
PLUS RISING AND CHILLING
COOKING TIME: ABOUT 1 HOUR

200ml (scant 1 cup) double cream
1 tablespoon caster sugar
1 quantity donut dough (see page 91)
groundnut oil, for deep-frying

Coffee custard base
6 egg yolks
150g (¾ cup) caster sugar, plus
2 tablespoons
100g (generous ¾ cup) plain flour
500ml (generous 2 cups) milk
2 tablespoons very strong coffee
1 vanilla pod, split lengthways

Coffee glaze
500g (4 cups) icing sugar
4 tablespoons very strong coffee
pinch of salt

❶ For the custard, place the egg yolks and sugar in a mixing bowl and whisk for 2 minutes until pale, then whisk in the flour thoroughly.

❷ Place the milk, coffee and vanilla pod in a small saucepan over a medium heat and bring to the boil. Pour the boiling milk over the egg yolk mixture and whisk until well combined.

❸ Pour the mixture back into the pan over a low heat and bring back to the boil, whisking all the time until very thick and smooth. Cover the surface with clingfilm to prevent a skin forming and leave to cool.

❹ Whip the cream with the remaining 2 tablespoons caster sugar until soft peaks form, then fold into the cooled custard. Refrigerate until ready to use.

❺ For the glaze, beat all the ingredients together until smooth. If it sets before using, gently warm to soften it again.

❻ Make the dough and cook the donuts following the instructions on page 91, rolling the dough out to about 1cm (½ inch) thick and cutting it into 10 x 4-cm (4 x 1½-inch) rectangles rather than cutting it into rings. Leave to cool for 30 minutes.

❼ Fit a piping bag with a plain nozzle large enough for the filling to pass through. Spoon the filling into the bag, insert the nozzle into each end of a cooked donut and squeeze until it plumps up slightly along its length. Repeat with the remaining donuts. Dip one side of each filled donut into the glaze and set on a wire rack, glaze-side up, until the glaze has set. Serve warm.

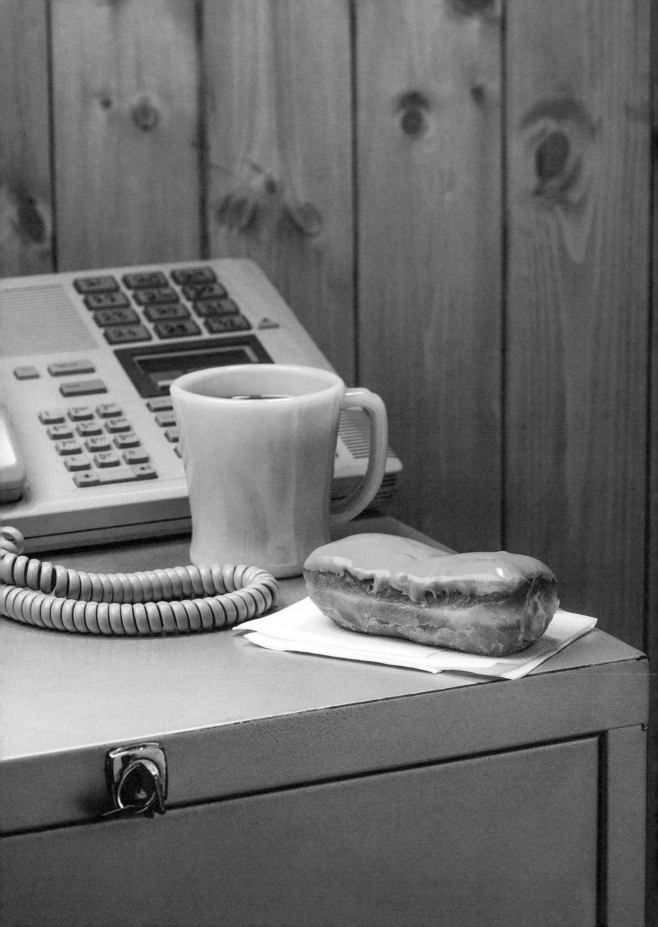

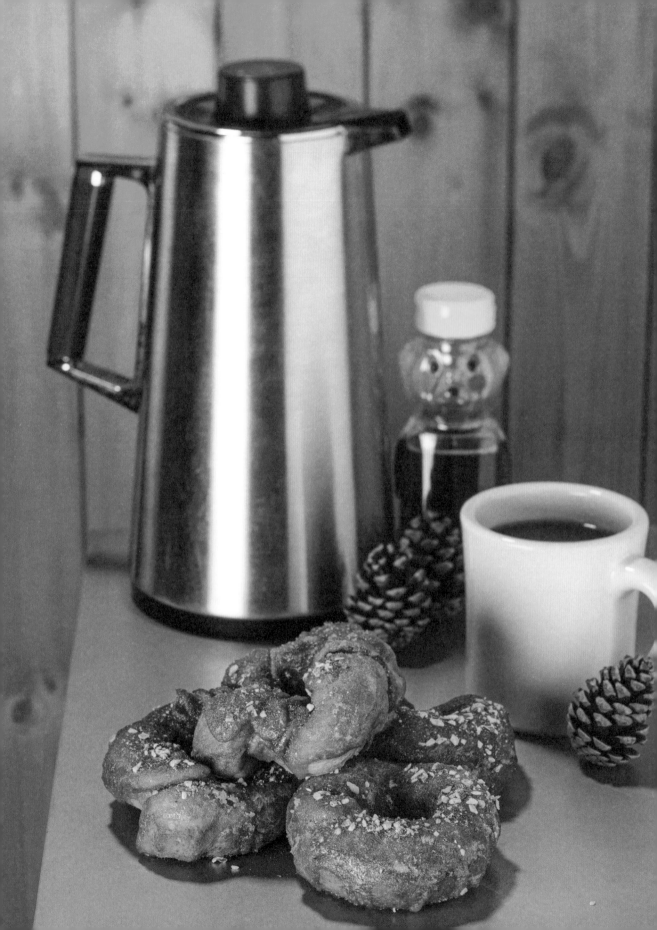

PUMPKIN DONUTS WITH VANILLA MAPLE GLAZE

MAKES 24
PREPARATION TIME: 2 HOURS,
PLUS OVERNIGHT FOR STARTER,
AND EXTRA FOR RISING
COOKING TIME: 45 MINUTES

1 quantity Sourdough Donut dough
(see page 100)

2 teaspoons ground cinnamon

1 teaspoon ground ginger

1 teaspoon ground nutmeg

½ teaspoon ground allspice

¼ teaspoon ground cloves

75g (⅓ cup) peeled, roasted pumpkin

50g (scant ¼ cup) light muscovado sugar

2 tablespoons pumpkin seeds

24 wafer-thin slices of pancetta or bacon
(optional)

groundnut oil, for deep-frying

butter, for greasing

Vanilla maple glaze

300g (1⅓ cups) light soft brown sugar

8 tablespoons maple syrup

1½ teaspoons vanilla extract

1½ tablespoons lemon juice

❶ Make the dough following steps 1–2 of the instructions on page 100, then knead in all of the spices until evenly incorporated. Mash the pumpkin flesh with the sugar and knead roughly into the dough, leaving a marbled effect.

❷ Divide the dough into 24 equal pieces and shape each piece into a ring. Arrange the donuts on a lightly greased tray, leaving space for them to expand. Lightly cover with greased clingfilm and leave in a warm place for 1–1½ hours or until doubled in size.

❸ Meanwhile, place the pumpkin seeds in a dry frying pan over a low–medium heat and toast for 8–10 minutes until golden. Transfer to a plate to cool, then crush to a fine powder using a pestle and mortar.

❹ When the donuts have risen, thread a slice of pancetta, if using, round each ring. To deep-fry, pour the oil into a large, deep saucepan or deep-fat fryer, making sure it is no more than one-third to one-half full. Heat the oil until it reaches 180°C (350°F) or until a cube of bread browns in 30 seconds.

❺ Carefully lower about 3 donuts at a time into the hot oil and fry for 2–3 minutes on each side until golden brown. Remove with a slotted spoon and drain on kitchen paper. Leave to cool a little.

❻ For the glaze, place the sugar, maple syrup and vanilla in a small saucepan over a low heat and stir gently until the sugar has dissolved. Remove from the heat and stir in the lemon juice. Dip the donuts into the glaze and sprinkle with the ground pumpkin seeds. Leave on a wire rack until the glaze has set. Serve warm.

GLAZED SOURDOUGH DONUTS

MAKES 24
PREPARATION TIME: 2 HOURS,
PLUS OVERNIGHT FOR STARTER,
AND EXTRA FOR RISING
COOKING TIME: 35 MINUTES

2 tablespoons active white wheat flour
sourdough starter

100ml (scant ½ cup) water

300g (scant 2¼ cups) strong white flour

3 tablespoons honey

50g (3½ tablespoons) butter, melted, plus
extra for greasing

100ml (scant ½ cup) milk

3 egg yolks, at room temperature

finely grated zest and juice of 1 small lemon

2 teaspoons fine sea salt

flour, for dusting

groundnut oil, for deep-frying

Glaze

300g (2 ½ cups) icing sugar

juice of 1–2 lemons

❶ The night before, mix 2 tablespoons of the sourdough starter with the water and 100g (¾ cup) of the flour. Cover and leave to ferment overnight, or until risen and bubbly on the surface. The next day, place the honey, butter and milk in a small saucepan over a low heat just until the butter has melted. Place the egg yolks in a small bowl with the lemon zest and juice and beat lightly. Mix the warm milk mixture with the active sourdough mixture (you should have about 250g/9oz), then add the egg yolk mixture and the remaining flour. Mix all the ingredients well to form a very soft, sticky dough. Wet your hands and scrape the dough on to a clean work surface.

❷ To knead the dough, lift each side up high to stretch it, then slap it back down on to the work surface, alternating from side to side. Continue for 15–20 minutes until the dough is elastic and has a smooth surface with bubbles forming under it. Cover and allow to rest for 20 minutes, then knead in the salt. Press out the dough on a lightly floured surface into a large rectangle, then fold up the bottom third into the middle, and the top third down on top. Cover and leave to rest for 30 minutes, then press out again, fold and rest 4 more times, allowing the dough to rest for 1 hour after the final folding.

❸ Stretch out the dough on a lightly floured surface to about 1cm (½ inch) thick. Use an 8-cm (3¼-inch) cutter to cut out rounds, then cut a hole out of the middle of each using a 3-cm (1¼-inch) cutter. Arrange the donuts on a lightly greased tray, leaving space for expansion. Cover with greased clingfilm and leave in a warm place for 1–1½ hours or until doubled in size.

❹ To deep-fry, pour the oil into a large, deep saucepan or deep-fat fryer, ensuring it is no more than one-third to one-half full. Heat the oil until it reaches 180°C (350°F), or until a cube of bread browns in 30 seconds. Carefully lower about 3 donuts at a time into the hot oil and fry for 2–3 minutes on each side until golden brown. Remove with a slotted spoon and drain on kitchen paper. Leave to cool a little. For the glaze, sieve the icing sugar into a bowl and add lemon juice to form a smooth, runny glaze. Dip the donuts into the glaze and set on a wire rack until the glaze has set. Serve warm.

PEANUT BUTTER DONUTS

MAKES 20
PREPARATION TIME: 1 HOUR 15 MINUTES, PLUS RISING AND CHILLING
COOKING TIME: ABOUT 35 MINUTES

1 quantity donut dough (see page 91)

groundnut oil, for deep-frying

sea salt flakes, for sprinkling

Peanut butter filling

100g (7 tablespoons) unsalted butter, softened

400g (generous 1½ cups) smooth peanut butter

100g (½ cup) icing sugar

pinch of sea salt

1½ teaspoons vanilla extract

400ml (1⅔ cups) double cream

Peanut butter glaze

500g (scant 4¼ cups) icing sugar

200–250ml (scant 1 cup–generous 1 cup) milk

200g (generous ¾ cup) smooth peanut butter

1½ teaspoons vanilla extract

1 For the filling, place the butter, peanut butter, icing sugar, salt and vanilla extract in a mixing bowl and beat until well combined.

2 Whip the cream until soft peaks form, then fold into the peanut butter mixture and refrigerate until ready to use.

3 For the glaze, beat all the ingredients together until smooth. If it sets before using, gently warm to soften it again.

4 Make the dough and cook the donuts following the instructions on page 91, rolling the dough into 20 balls about the size of a golf ball rather than cutting it into rings. Leave to cool for 30 minutes.

5 Fit a piping bag with a plain nozzle large enough for the filling to pass through. Spoon the filling into the bag, insert the nozzle into the side of a cooked donut and squeeze until it plumps up slightly. Repeat with the remaining donuts. Dip each filled donut into the glaze and sprinkle with a few sea salt flakes. Leave on a wire rack until the glaze has set.

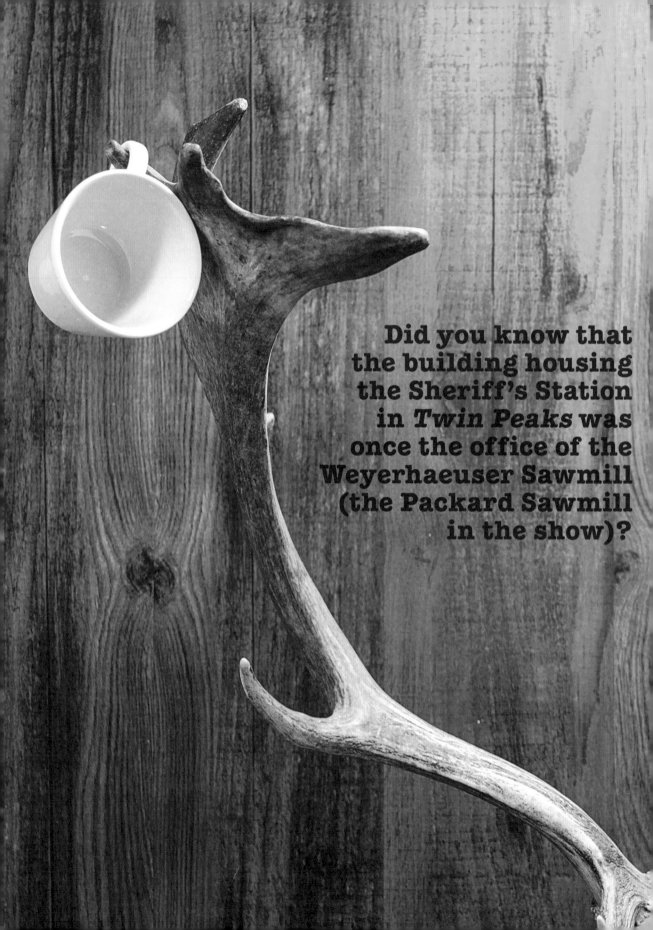

Did you know that the building housing the Sheriff's Station in *Twin Peaks* was once the office of the Weyerhaeuser Sawmill (the Packard Sawmill in the show)?

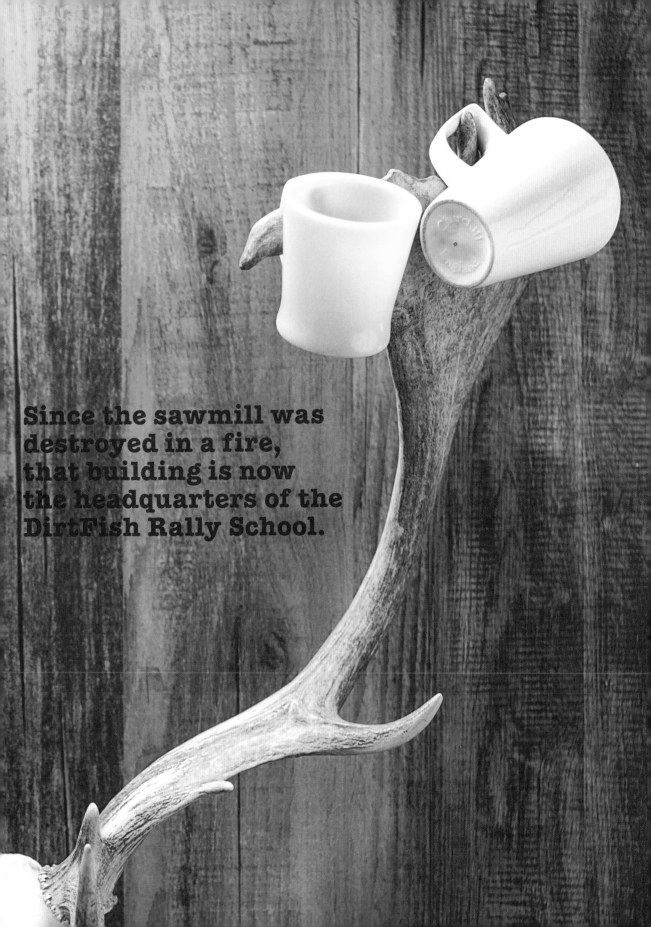

Since the sawmill was
destroyed in a fire,
that building is now
the headquarters of the
DirtFish Rally School.

HAWK'S CHOCOLATE DECADENCE DONUTS

MAKES 20
**PREPARATION TIME: 1 HOUR, PLUS
RISING AND CHILLING**
COOKING TIME: ABOUT 35 MINUTES

1 quantity donut dough (see page 91),
made with 4 tablespoons cocoa powder
replacing 4 tablespoons of the flour

50g (⅓ cup) chocolate chips

groundnut oil, for deep-frying

Chocolate glaze

600ml (2½ cups) double cream

300g (1¾ cups) plain dark chocolate
(minimum 70% cocoa solids), broken
into cubes

120g (generous ⅔ cup) milk chocolate,
broken into cubes

pinch of salt

❶ Make the dough and cook the donuts following the
instructions on page 91, kneading the chocolate chips into
the dough before rolling out and cutting into rings. Leave to
cool for 30 minutes.

❷ For the glaze, place the cream in a small saucepan over
a low heat. Bring to the boil, then remove from the heat. Add
the chocolate and salt and stir until melted and smooth. Dip
the donuts into the glaze while the glaze is still warm and
leave on a wire rack until the glaze has set. Serve warm.

CONTRIBUTED BY
CAST MEMBER
AL STROBEL

PECAN CRESCENTS

MAKES 50
PREPARATION TIME: 30 MINUTES
COOKING TIME: 25–30 MINUTES

250g (2¼ sticks) butter, softened

4 tablespoons icing sugar, plus extra for dusting

2 teaspoons vanilla extract

200g (1¾ cups) ground pecans

300g (scant 2½ cups) plain flour

½ teaspoon salt

1 Preheat the oven to 160°C (325°F), Gas Mark 3 and line 2 baking sheets with baking parchment.

2 Place the butter in a large mixing bowl and beat until smooth. Beat in the remaining ingredients.

3 Divide the mixture into 50 equal pieces, then shape each piece into a crescent moon.

4 Arrange the cookies on the lined baking sheets and cook for 25–30 minutes until lightly golden. Dust with a little icing sugar and cool on a wire rack.

The station wagon that Al Strobel (AKA Mike) drives in *Fire Walk With Me* is actually his own vehicle. He thought his vehicle suited the film a lot better than the original car that was to be used. He still drives the same station wagon to this day.

THE LOG LADY'S SUGAR COOKIES

MAKES 16–18
PREPARATION TIME: 15 MINUTES
COOKING TIME: 15–20 MINUTES

250g (2 cups) plain flour, plus extra for dusting

150g (1⅜ sticks) unsalted butter, cubed

125g (generous ½ cup) caster sugar

1 teaspoon vanilla extract

pinch of salt

❶ Preheat the oven to 160°C (325°F), Gas Mark 3 and line 2 baking sheets with baking parchment.

❷ Place the flour in a mixing bowl, add the butter and rub in with the fingertips until the mixture resembles fine breadcrumbs. Stir in the sugar, vanilla extract and salt and bring the mixture together into a smooth ball.

❸ Roll out the dough on a lightly floured surface to about 7mm (⅜ inch) thick and cut into 8-cm (3¼-inch) rounds using a fluted cookie cutter.

❹ Arrange the cookies on the lined baking sheets and cook for 15–20 minutes until lightly golden. Cool on a wire rack.

The Log Lady was an idea formed in David Lynch's mind long before *Twin Peaks*. As far back as *Eraserhead*, he and Catherine E. Coulson were discussing the character.

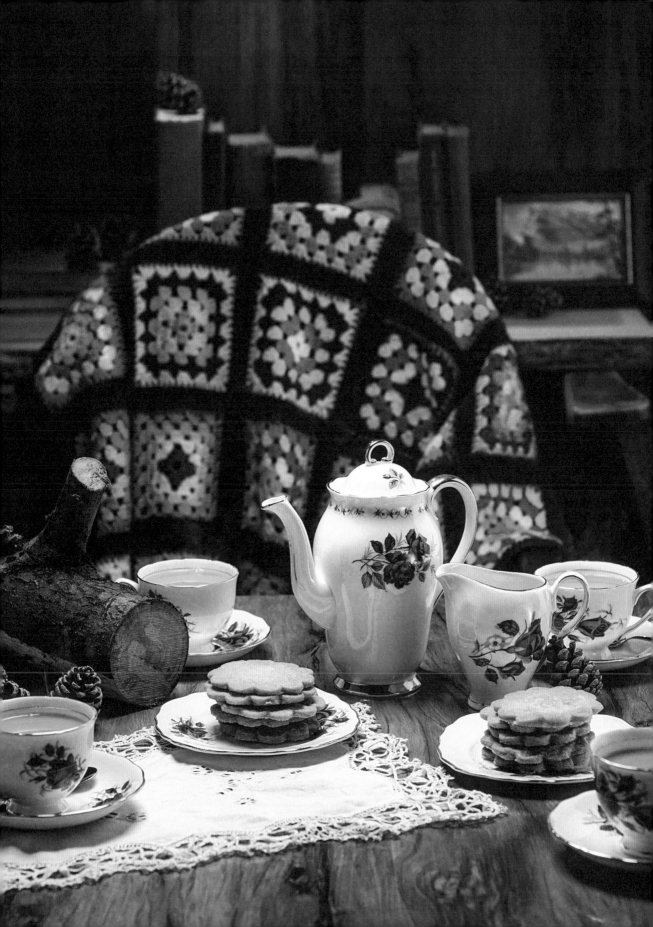

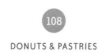

MERINGUE BLONDIES WITH BOOZY CHERRIES

SERVES 6
PREPARATION TIME: 10 MINUTES
COOKING TIME: 10–12 MINUTES

2 large egg whites

100g (½ cup) caster sugar

6 shop-bought blondies or thick slices of plain cake

150g (5½oz) canned pitted black cherries in syrup, drained

Boozy cherries

150g (5½oz) canned pitted black cherries in syrup, drained

1 teaspoon finely grated lemon zest

2 teaspoons lemon juice

3 tablespoons kirsch or cherry brandy

75g (generous ⅓ cup) caster sugar

❶ Preheat the oven to 180°C (350°F), Gas Mark 4 and line a large baking sheet with baking parchment. Whisk the egg whites and sugar in a clean bowl until the mixture forms soft peaks.

❷ Place the blondies or cake slices on the prepared baking sheet and pile the cherries on to the cakes. Spoon the meringue mixture over the cherries in attractive peaks. Bake for 10–12 minutes until pale golden.

❸ For the boozy cherries, place all the ingredients in a saucepan and heat gently, stirring occasionally, until the sugar has dissolved. Increase the heat and simmer gently for 5–6 minutes until slightly syrupy. Spoon the mixture into 6 serving dishes.

❹ Arrange the blondies on top of the boozy cherries and serve immediately.

SARAH PALMER'S CAPPUCCINO COOKIES

MAKES ABOUT 20
PREPARATION TIME: 20 MINUTES
COOKING TIME: 10–15 MINUTES

225g (2 sticks) unsalted butter, softened

75g (generous ½ cup) icing sugar, sifted

½ teaspoon vanilla extract

200g (scant 1⅔ cups) plain flour

4 tablespoons cornflour

1–2 tablespoons milk

1 tablespoon cocoa powder

1 teaspoon coffee essence

hot chocolate powder, for dusting

1 Preheat the oven to 200°C (400°F), Gas Mark 6 and line 2 large baking sheets with baking parchment.

2 Place the butter, icing sugar and vanilla extract in a bowl and beat together with a hand-held electric whisk until light and fluffy. Sift in the flour and cornflour and stir until smooth, adding just enough of the milk to form a dough of piping consistency.

3 Place half of the mixture in a second bowl, sift in the cocoa powder and fold in until combined. Stir the coffee essence into the first bowl until evenly combined.

4 Spoon the cocoa mixture into one side of a piping bag fitted with a star-shaped nozzle, and the coffee-flavoured mixture into the other side so that both mixtures will be piped out at the same time. Pipe about 20 whirls or other shapes on to the prepared baking sheets.

5 Bake for 10–15 minutes until lightly golden, then transfer to wire racks to cool. Serve dusted with chocolate powder.

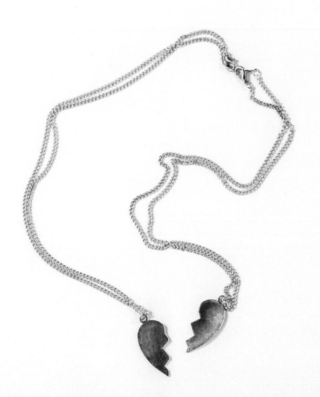

chapter 4

WHITE LODGE FAMILY DINING

THE WHITE LODGE

As Major Briggs reveals, the doors to the Black and White Lodge are opened by fear and love. Although the White Lodge does not feature in *Twin Peaks* as heavily as the Black Lodge, what is revealed creates an image of love, purity, goodness and honesty. The White Lodge is, in fact, still quite a mystery in the world of *Twin Peaks*.

You could speculate that the White Lodge is the antithesis of the Black Lodge. For each corrupted doppleganger in the Black Lodge, you could imagine one pure of heart in the White Lodge. Deputy Hawk explains that his people believe the White Lodge is place where spirits reside and he could be right. But

essentially the White Lodge is whatever your mind decides it is.

In this section, I wanted to bring you good, wholesome food. The kind of food you can imagine any of the *Twin Peaks* matriarchs cooking up for their family. When you think of *Twin Peaks* family dining and conversations around the table, you may conjure up love when it comes to the Hayward family, unhappiness when it comes to the Hornes, and deception when it comes to the Palmers. But one thing links them all…secrets, they're filled with secrets.

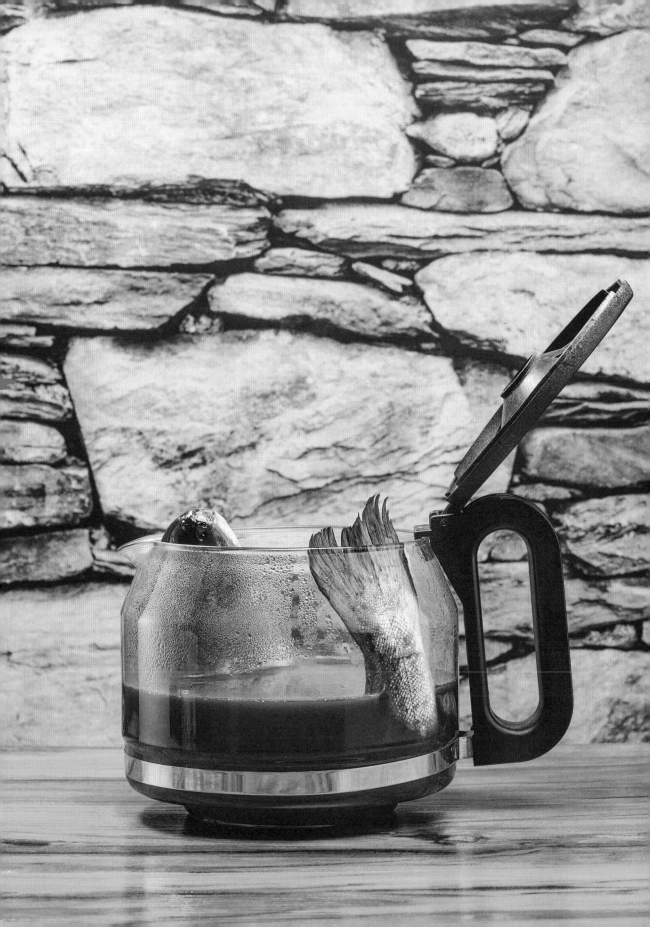

PERCOLATOR FISH SUPPER

SERVES 4
PREPARATION TIME: 15 MINUTES
COOKING TIME: 20 MINUTES

75g (5 tablespoons) butter

2 garlic cloves, crushed

75ml (⅓ cup) bourbon whiskey

200ml (scant 1 cup) very strong coffee

2 teaspoons brown sugar

1½ tablespoons lemon or lime juice

4 whole trout, about 400g (14oz) each, gutted

salt and pepper

To garnish

25g (2 tablespoons) butter

100g (scant 1 cup) pecans or almonds, sliced lengthways

3 tablespoons chopped parsley

❶ Place the butter and garlic in a saucepan over a high heat until foaming. Add the bourbon, let it bubble up then add the coffee and sugar. Bring to the boil, lower the heat and simmer for 3–4 minutes, or until reduced by half. Add the lemon juice and season with salt and pepper.

❷ Preheat the grill to hot. Season the trout inside and out, slash the flesh 3 times on each side and arrange on a baking sheet. Spoon a little sauce evenly over the fish and cook under the grill for about 5 minutes until golden. Carefully turn the fish, spoon over more sauce and cook for a further 5–6 minutes or until cooked through.

❸ For the garnish, place the butter in a frying pan over a medium heat, add the nuts and cook for 3–4 minutes, stirring occasionally, until lightly toasted. Stir in the chopped parsley and spoon over the trout to serve.

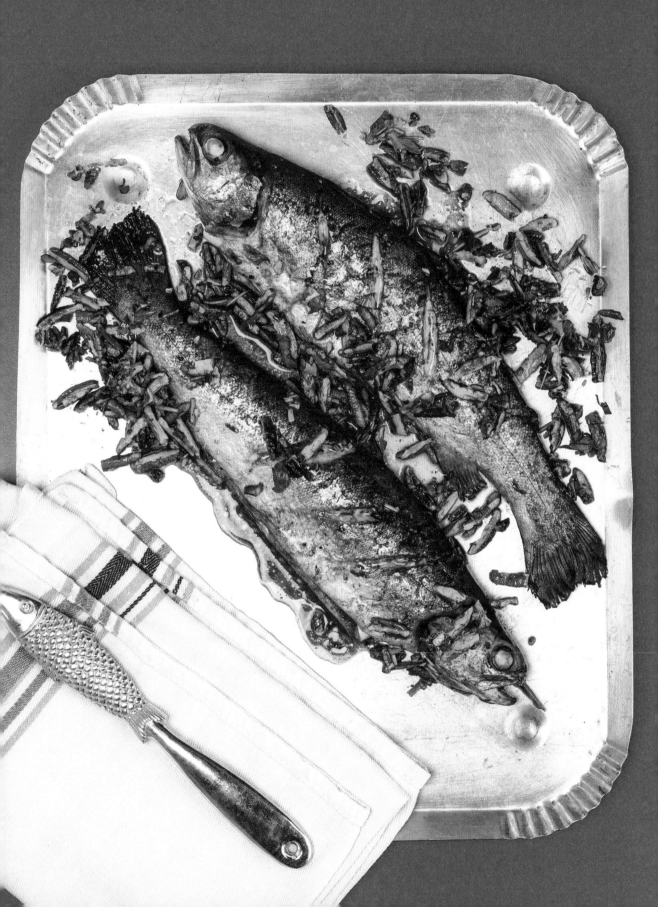

BETTY BRIGGS'S NUT LOAF

SERVES 6–8
PREPARATION TIME: 1 HOUR
COOKING TIME: 2 HOURS

2 tablespoons olive oil, plus extra
for greasing

300g (10½oz) cavolo nero or other cabbage
leaves, thick stems removed

50g (scant ½ cup) pecans, crushed

50g (scant ½ cup) hazelnuts, crushed

50g (scant ½ cup) cashews, crushed

50g (¼ cup) wild and white rice mix

1 onion, chopped

3 garlic cloves, sliced

1 red chilli, deseeded and finely chopped

leaves from 1 large thyme sprig

150g (generous 1 cup) canned or vac-packed
chestnuts, crushed

250g (2½ cups) portobello mushrooms,
chopped

finely grated zest and juice of 1 lemon

2 tablespoons chopped tarragon leaves

60g (generous 1 cup) fresh breadcrumbs

50g (scant ½ cup) dried cranberries

3 tablespoons chopped parsley

50g (½ cup) Pecorino or Parmesan cheese,
finely grated

3 large eggs

200ml (scant 1 cup) crème fraîche

salt and pepper

❶ For the sauce, preheat the oven to 200°C (400°F), Gas Mark 6. Spread the almonds out a baking sheet and toast in the oven for 5–10 minutes until golden brown. Set aside.

❷ Place the peppers, garlic, tomatoes and chilli on a baking sheet. Drizzle with a little of the olive oil, season with salt and pepper, toss to coat and cook in the oven for about 30 minutes, or until all the vegetables are tender and lightly charred.

❸ Meanwhile, heat 3 tablespoons of the olive oil in a frying pan over a high heat and fry the bread until golden brown on both sides.

❹ Remove the vegetables from the oven and leave to cool a little, then peel off all the skins and remove the seeds and stalks from the peppers and chilli. Squeeze the flesh from the garlic skins.

❺ Place the almonds, fried bread and roasted garlic in a food processor and blend to a smooth paste. Add the remaining roasted vegetables and blend to a cream, then gradually add the vinegar and the remaining olive oil. Season to taste and set aside until ready to serve.

❻ For the nut loaf, preheat the oven to 180°C (350°F), Gas Mark 4 and grease a 1.5-litre (2½-pint) loaf tin. Blanch the cabbage leaves in a large saucepan of lightly salted boiling water until just tender. Drain, refresh in cold water and drain well again. Use the leaves to line the loaf tin.

Romesco sauce

100g (scant ⅔ cup) almonds

2 small red or Romano peppers, about 250g (9oz) in total

4 garlic cloves, unpeeled

3–4 ripe tomatoes, about 400g (14oz) in total

1 fresh red chilli

300ml (1¼ cups) olive oil

50g (1 cup) white bread without crusts, cubed

1 tablespoon wine vinegar

7 Spread all the nuts on a baking sheet and toast in the oven for about 10 minutes or until golden. Cook the rice according to the packet instructions in a large saucepan of lightly salted boiling water until tender. Drain and set aside.

8 Heat the olive oil in a large frying pan over a medium heat, add the onion, garlic, chilli and thyme and cook gently, without colouring, for 5–6 minutes or until softened. Add the chestnuts, mushrooms, lemon zest and tarragon and cook, stirring occasionally, for 10–15 minutes until the mushrooms are tender and any moisture has evaporated. Stir in the lemon juice and season to taste.

9 Transfer the mixture to a large bowl, then stir in the rice, breadcrumbs, cranberries, parsley and nuts. Beat the Pecorino, eggs and crème fraîche together until smooth, stir into the mushroom mixture and season to taste. Scrape the mixture into the prepared loaf tin and bake for 45–50 minutes or until just set. Turn out, slice and serve accompanied by the Romesco sauce.

See photograph overleaf.

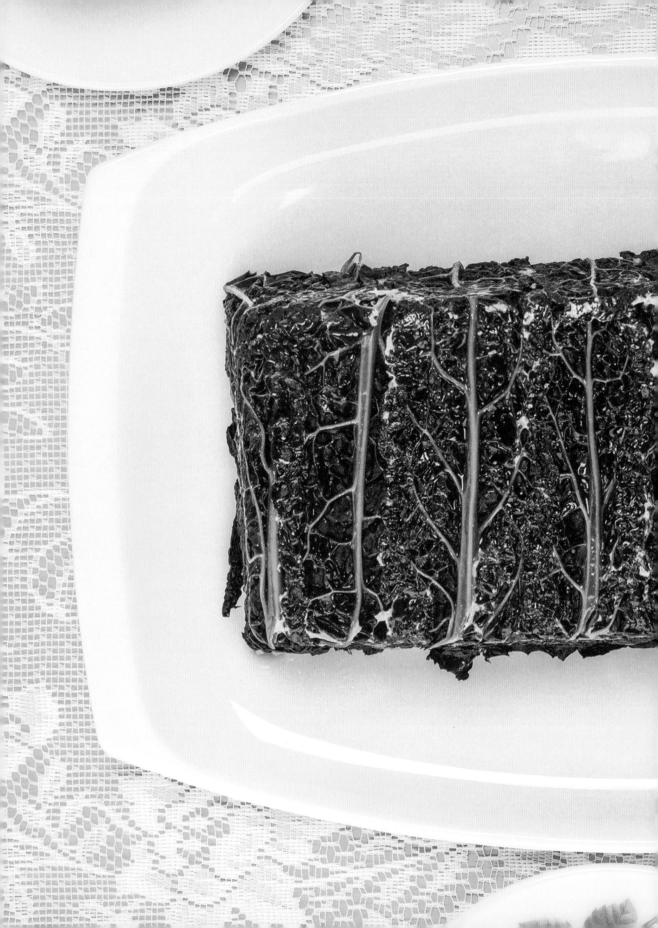

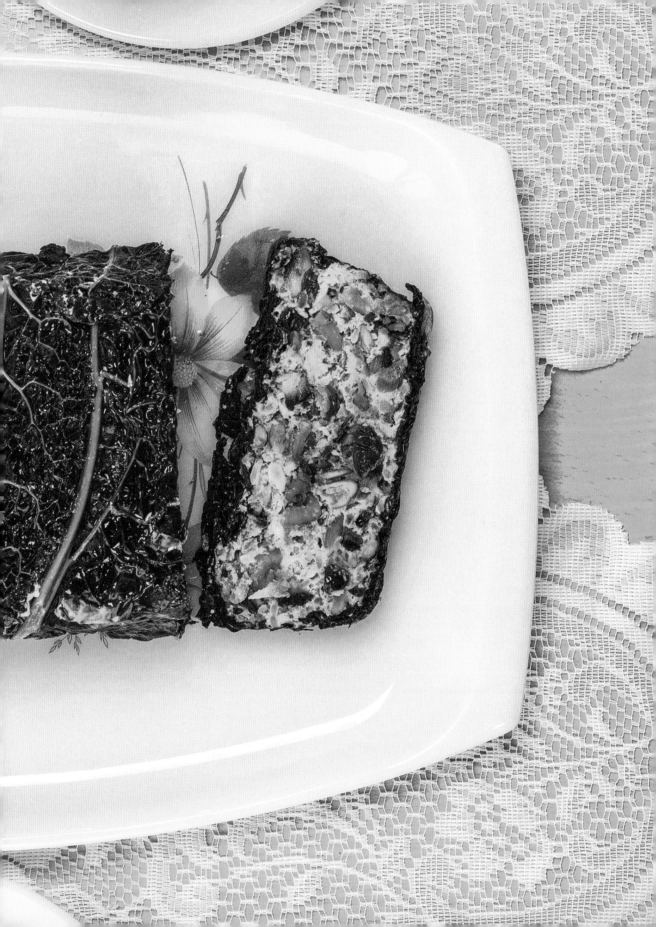

DOC HAYWARD'S "DIET" LASAGNE

SERVES 6
PREPARATION TIME: 30 MINUTES
COOKING TIME: 1 HOUR 15 MINUTES

650g (1lb 7oz) peeled pumpkin,
cut into large cubes

8 tablespoons olive oil

250g (9oz) cherry tomatoes

2 aubergines, thinly sliced lengthways

2 tablespoons sage leaves, stalks removed

150g (1½ cups) Parmesan cheese,
finely grated

250g (generous 1 cup) ricotta

½ teaspoon ground nutmeg

4 tablespoons milk

250g (generous 1 cup) mascarpone

100g (1 cup) mozzarella, grated

salt and pepper

❶ Preheat the oven to 200°C (400°F), Gas Mark 6. Arrange the pumpkin cubes on a baking sheet, drizzle with 2 tablespoons of the olive oil, season well and cook for 15 minutes. Add the cherry tomatoes to the baking sheet and return to the oven for 10–15 minutes or until the pumpkin is tender when pierced by a knife. Set aside to cool.

❷ Lay the aubergine slices in a single layer on 2–3 baking sheets and brush with 4 tablespoons of the remaining oil. Season and bake for 15–20 minutes until tender and golden. Set aside.

❸ Heat the remaining oil in a large frying pan over a high heat and add the sage leaves. As they crisp up, remove with a slotted spoon and drain on kitchen paper.

❹ Once the pumpkin is cool, place in a bowl, mash well and stir in two-thirds of the grated Parmesan, the ricotta and nutmeg and season well with salt and pepper.

❺ Spread a layer of the pumpkin mixture in the bottom of an ovenproof dish. Scatter with a few of the roasted tomatoes and sage leaves, then add a layer of aubergine slices. Continue with the layers to use up the remaining ingredients, finishing with a layer of aubergine.

❻ Place the milk in a bowl with the mascarpone and remaining Parmesan, season and beat to combine. Pour over the lasagne, sprinkle the mozzarella evenly over the surface and bake for 25–30 minutes, or until bubbling and heated through.

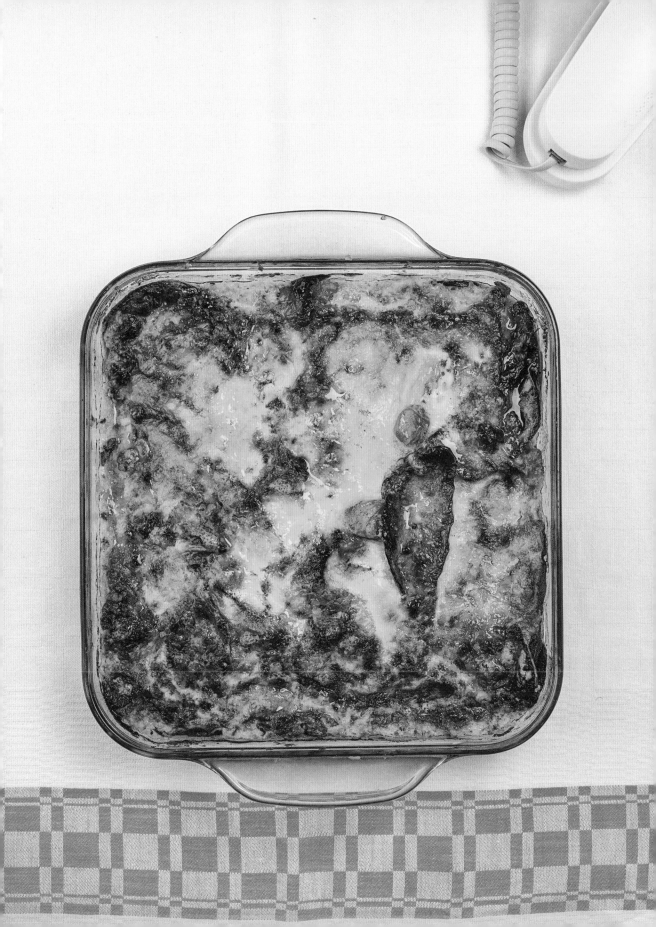

LUDO INSPIRED BY TWIN PEAKS

Those of us who watched *Twin Peaks* the first time round are old enough to remember the infamous *Twin Peaks* board game which was released in 1991.

Every now and then one of these games pops up on eBay, but they are now collectors' items and the price reflects this. So rather than play that game, we thought we would put a little Peaky twist on the classic board game, Ludo. Enjoy!

HOW TO MAKE A LUDO BOARD

All Ludo boards follow the same basic design and this one's no different.

You will need

1 piece of card 30cm (12 inches) square

4 pictures of items that are reminiscent of *Twin Peaks*

ruler

permanent marker

coloured pens or pencils

glue

The method

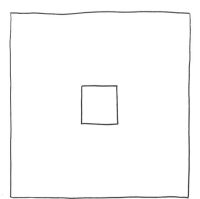

❶ Find the very centre of the piece of card and draw a square – that is your home square. Try to make it as central as possible so the rest of the board is symmetrical.

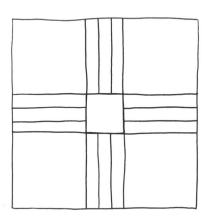

❷ Continue the sides of the square out to the edges of the card to make a large cross shape. Divide each arm of the cross into 3 equal columns, leaving the home square clear.

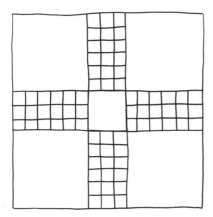

❸ Now divide each column into 6 equal squares. You will end up with 18 squares in each arm of the cross, 72 in total.

❹ Write "Home" in the home square, in the centre of the board. Next glue the 4 pictures into the large squares. It is up to you what pictures you use for inspiration.

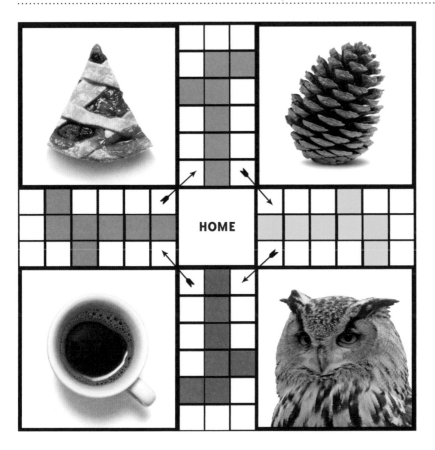

❺ Using coloured pens or pencils, colour in 6 of the squares on each arm, as shown in the illustration. The arms should each have squares of a different colour.

HOW TO MAKE THE CHARACTERS

You now have your *Twin Peaks*-inspired Ludo board, so now you need to make your characters.

You will need

16 strips of card, about 10 x 2cm (4 x ¾ inch)

glue

16 pictures of *Twin Peaks* characters, about 2cm (¾ inch) square, 2 copies of each

16 paperclips

The method

Each of your four pictures needs four characters associated with it (for example, Agent Dale Cooper for the cherry pie, BOB for the owl). You need two pictures of each character, one for each side of its counter.

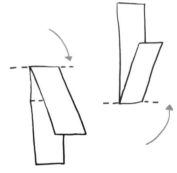

❶ Take a strip of card. Make a fold across it about 4cm (1⅝ inch) from each end, pressing the creases down well. Turn the strip of card over.

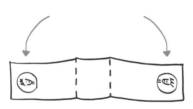

❷ Take a character picture and glue it to one end of the strip of card, with the top of the head towards the edge. Repeat with its doppelganger at the other end of the strip. Repeat for the remaining characters and pieces of card.

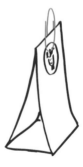

❸ When the glue is dry, pinch the two ends of the strip of card together, glue in place and hold securely with a paperclip. They should stand up on their flat bases.

How to play

Now you are ready to play *Twin Peaks*-inspired Ludo! Not sure how to play? Here's the rules...

Ludo can be played with 2–4 players. Each player must pick a picture and four characters associated with that picture. The object of the game is for all your four characters to start at their picture, travel around the board, and make it back to the home square in the middle of the board. The player whose four characters reach the home square first wins.

❶ Each player must throw a 6 to start. They can then move their first character on to the first coloured square next to their picture. They then have another throw and can proceed forward by the number of squares on the dice. The characters move around the board in a clockwise fashion, following the outline of the cross shape by moving along the white squares round the outside of the cross.

❷ At each subsequent throw of a 6, a player can bring a fresh character into play, or may choose to advance a character who is already moving round the board. Throwing a 6 always entitles a player to a second throw.

❸ When a character lands on a space occupied by another player's character, it takes its place and sends the first character back to its picture, from where it has to start its journey again (throwing a 6 to leave the picture square).

❹ When two or more of a player's characters land on the same space, they form a barrier which no other player's character may seize or overtake. If a player's character cannot pass another player's barrier then their turn is lost.

❺ When a character has travelled one lap of the board and is back to its picture square, it then follows the coloured squares up to the home square. To reach the home square, the exact number of moves must be thrown. If the player throws a higher number than the moves needed, the character must travel back down the coloured squares and keep trying until he gets home. The winner of the game is the player who gets all four of his characters home first!

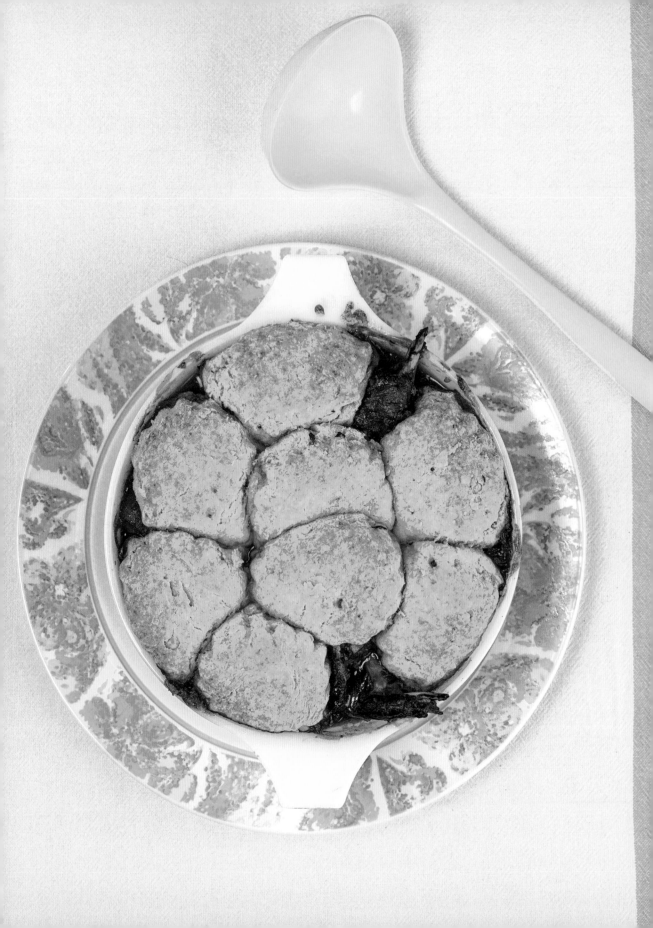

BIG ED'S ROADSIDE STEW

SERVES 4
PREPARATION TIME: 45 MINUTES
COOKING TIME: 2–3 HOURS

50g (generous ⅓ cup) plain flour

2 prepared rabbits, each jointed into 6

3 tablespoons olive oil

5 red onions, thickly sliced

2 large garlic cloves, crushed

1 teaspoon fennel seeds, crushed

500ml (generous 2 cups) dark beer

1 litre (4¼ cups) chicken stock

300g (10½oz) baby carrots

pared rind from 1 lemon

3 bay leaves

1 star anise

salt and pepper

Buttermilk biscuits

300g (scant 2½ cups) plain flour, plus extra for dusting

1 teaspoon salt

2 teaspoons baking powder

½ teaspoon bicarbonate of soda

150g (1⅜ sticks) butter, cubed

2 tablespoons chopped tarragon

280ml (scant 1¼ cups) buttermilk or milk

❶ For the stew, tip the flour on to a large plate, season well and dip the rabbit pieces in it to coat all over. Heat the oil in a large, ovenproof casserole over a high heat and add the rabbit, a few pieces at a time, turning regularly until browned on all sides. Transfer the rabbit pieces to a plate and set aside.

❷ Reduce the heat under the pan, add the onions, garlic and fennel seeds and cook gently for 10–15 minutes or until very soft. Preheat the oven to 150°C (300°F), Gas Mark 2.

❸ Pour the beer into the pan and let it bubble up. Add the stock and return the rabbit pieces to the pan with the carrots, lemon rind, bay leaves and star anise. Season, bring to the boil, cover and bake for 2–3 hours or until the meat is very tender.

❹ For the biscuits, place the flour, salt, baking powder and bicarbonate of soda in a large bowl and mix well. Rub the butter into the dry ingredients until the mixture resembles fine breadcrumbs. Add the tarragon, then lightly mix in the buttermilk or milk to form a soft dough, being careful not to overmix it.

❺ Turn out on to a lightly floured surface and press the dough out with your fingertips to about 1cm (½ inch) thick. Use a plain cookie cutter to cut the dough into 6-cm (2½-inch) rounds. Roll up the scraps and use to make more biscuits.

❻ When the stew is almost ready, increase the oven temperature to 180°C (350°F), Gas Mark 4. Uncover the stew and arrange the biscuits on top. Cook the stew for a further 30–35 minutes or until the biscuits are golden. Serve immediately.

NORWEGIAN MEATBALLS & GRAVY

SERVES 6
PREPARATION TIME: 15 MINUTES
COOKING TIME: 30 MINUTES

250g (generous 1 cup) minced pork

250g (generous 1 cup) minced veal or beef

2½ tablespoons potato or plain flour

½ teaspoon ground ginger

¼ teaspoon ground nutmeg

¼ teaspoon ground allspice

½ teaspoon pepper

1½ teaspoons salt

150ml (⅔ cup) milk

50g (3½ tablespoons) butter

300ml (1¼ cups) beef or chicken stock

200ml (scant 1 cup) double cream or crème fraîche

50g (½ cup) Brunost, Gjetost or other semi-hard goats' cheese, grated (optional)

pinch of cayenne pepper or paprika

mashed potatoes, to serve

1 Place the minced meat in a large bowl with all the spices and seasoning. Gradually beat in the milk until the mixture forms a thick paste. Spoon out small nuggets of the meat mixture and form into rough ovals in the palm of your hand.

2 Melt half the butter in a heavy-based frying pan over a medium heat. Add half the meatballs and cook them for 5–6 minutes, turning occasionally, until lightly browned on all sides. Transfer to a plate and repeat with the remaining butter and meatballs. Set the meatballs aside.

3 Place the pan back on the heat and add the stock. Bring to the boil, lower the heat and simmer until reduced by half. Add the cream and simmer for a few minutes more until thickened.

4 Return the meatballs to the frying pan and simmer for 3–4 minutes until cooked through. Stir in the grated cheese (if using), season to taste and add a pinch of cayenne. Serve with the gravy and mashed potatoes.

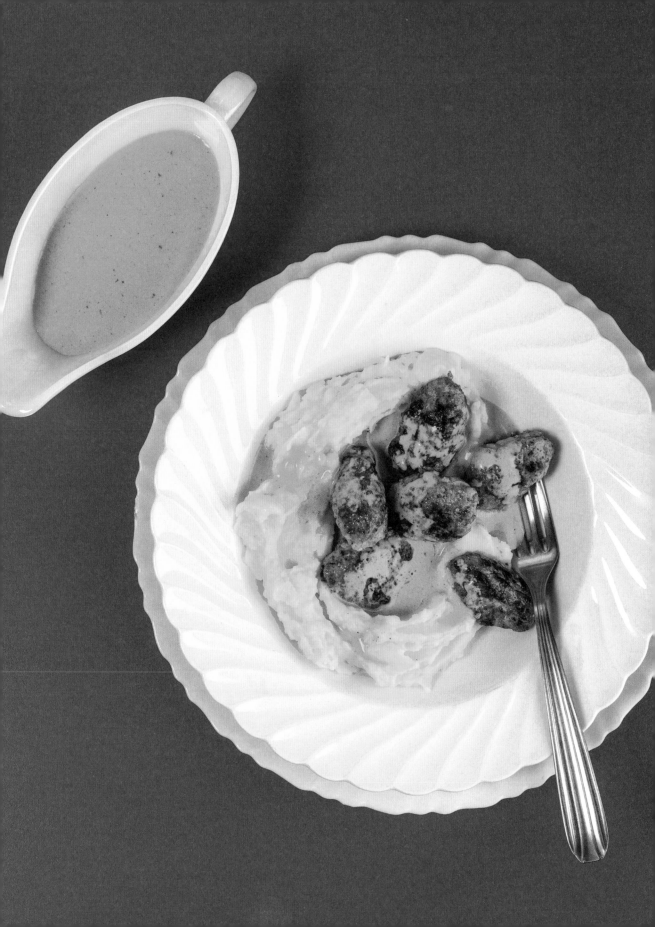

ICELANDIC HANGIKJOT

SERVES 6–8
PREPARATION TIME: DAYS 1, 2, AND 3:
10 MINUTES; 48 HOURS; 25 MINUTES
COOKING TIME: 1 HOUR 10 MINUTES –
1 HOUR 25 MINUTES, PLUS RESTING

6 litres (5¼ quarts) water

600g (scant 1¾ cups) honey

400g (1⅓ cups) sea salt, plus an extra
pinch for the potatoes

20 bay leaves

6 whole heads of garlic, smashed

125g (4½oz) mint, including stems,
roughly chopped

2.5kg (5lb 8oz) leg of lamb

1kg (2lb 4oz) potatoes, thickly sliced

2–3 tablespoons olive oil

pinch of sea salt

few sprigs of thyme

bunches of rosemary and bay leaves,
to garnish

salt and pepper

You will also need

200g (7oz) wood chips (use fruit or nut
woods, such as cherry, apple, almond,
pecan or hickory

❶ Place one-third of the measured water in a large saucepan
with the honey, salt and bay leaves and garlic and heat gently
for a few minutes, stirring occasionally, until the salt has
dissolved. Remove from the heat, add the remaining water
and stir in the chopped mint, then leave to cool completely.

❷ Pierce the lamb all over with a small knife to help the
brine permeate the meat, then place it in a deep, non-
metallic container. Pour the brine over the lamb and use a
large saucepan lid or other weight to hold the meat under
the brine if it bobs to the surface. It should be completely
submerged. Place in a cool place for at least 48 hours.

❸ When ready to cook, drain the lamb well, then season
all over with salt and pepper. Line a large, heavy-based
roasting tin with a double layer of aluminium foil. Scatter
evenly with the wood chips. Either lay another layer of foil
on top, turning up the edges slightly to catch any drips of fat
or juice from the lamb, or sit a second smaller roasting tin
on top of the woodchips.

❹ Place a small metal trivet on top of the foil or tin and lay
the lamb on top. Create a large lid with more foil, leaving
enough room for air to circulate inside, and seal very tightly
around the edges of the tin.

❺ Place the roasting tin on the stove over a high heat for
5 minutes (the contents will start to smoke at this point).
Reduce the heat to medium–low and continue to smoke
for 40 minutes. Remove the tin from the heat.

6 Preheat the oven to 220°C (425°F), Gas Mark 7. Remove the foil lid from the roasting tin, lift out the lamb on its trivet, and then carefully remove the drip foil or tin and set it aside. Next remove the remaining foil and woodchips from the tin and wipe it clean.

7 Pour the juices from smoking the lamb into the bottom of the cleaned roasting tin. Tip the sliced potatoes into the bottom of the tin with the olive oil, a pinch of sea salt and the thyme sprigs. Toss together well, then place the lamb on its trivet on top of the potatoes.

8 Place the roasting tin in the oven and roast the contents for 10 minutes. Reduce the heat to 180°C (350°F), Gas Mark 4, and roast for a further 15 minutes for rare or 10–15 minutes for medium to well done.

9 Remove the roasting tin from the oven, cover with aluminium foil and leave to rest for 15 minutes before serving on a large platter on a bed of rosemary and bay leaves.

See photograph overleaf.

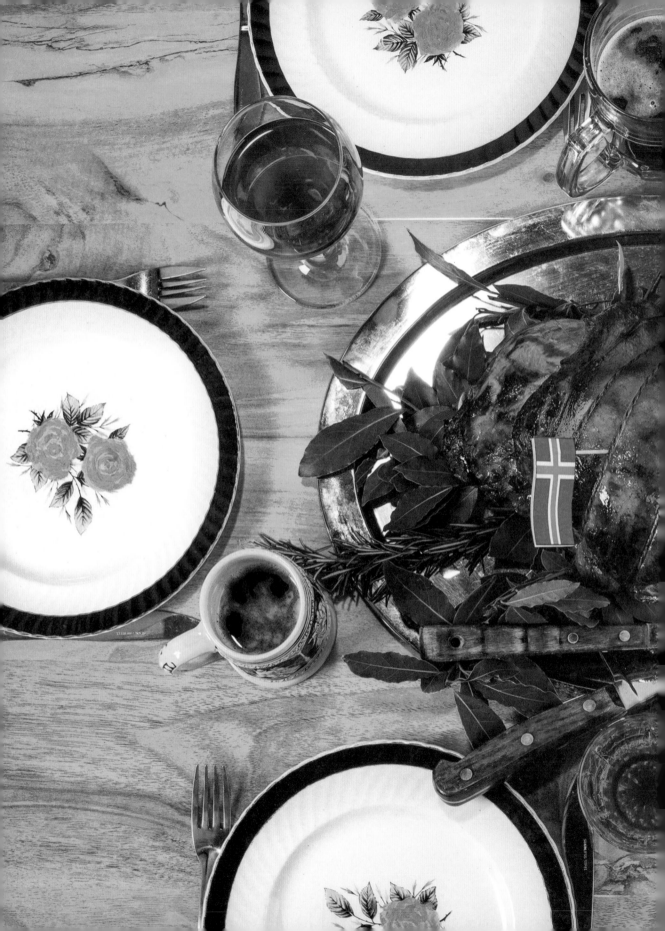

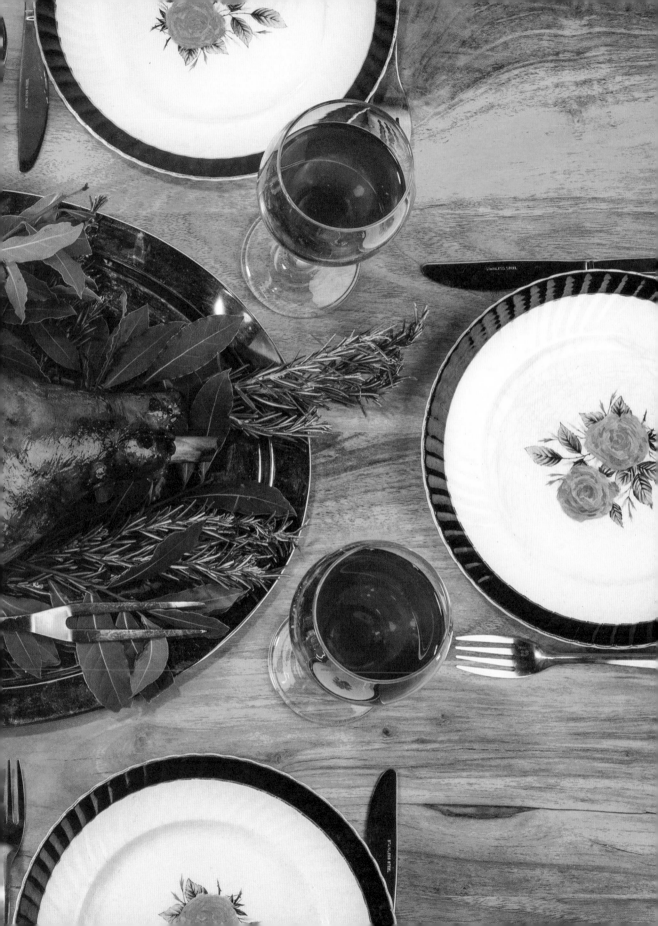

MAC 'N' CHEESE

SERVES 4–6
PREPARATION TIME: 30 MINUTES
COOKING TIME: 1 HOUR

450ml (scant 2 cups) double cream

450ml (scant 2 cups) milk

2 tablespoons chopped basil leaves, stalks reserved

50g (3½ tablespoons) butter

4 heaped tablespoons flour

150ml (⅔ cup) crème fraîche

½ teaspoon grated nutmeg

500g (5 cups) dried macaroni or spiralli

100g (1 cup) pecans, chopped

2 garlic cloves, crushed

50g (1 cup) day-old bread, crumbled

50g (½ cup) Parmesan cheese, finely grated

100ml (scant ½ cup) avocado oil or extra virgin olive oil

200g (2 cups) mozzarella, grated

150g (⅔ cup) peeled, roasted pumpkin, mashed

salt and pepper

green salad, to serve

❶ Pour the cream and milk into a small saucepan over a medium heat and add the basil stalks. Bring almost to the boil, then remove from the heat. Cover the pan and leave to infuse for a few minutes.

❷ Melt the butter in a large, heavy-based saucepan, add the flour and cook for 1–2 minutes. Discard the basil stalks, then carefully whisk in the warmed milk mixture, a little at a time, to make a smooth sauce. Stir in the crème fraîche and nutmeg and season well. Cover and set aside.

❸ Cook the pasta in a large saucepan of lightly salted boiling water according to the packet instructions until just tender. Drain well. Preheat the oven 200°C (400°F), Gas Mark 6.

❹ Place the pecans in a bowl with the garlic, bread, chopped basil and one-third of the grated Parmesan. Add the oil and mix well.

❺ Stir the pasta into the white sauce with half the mozzarella, the remaining Parmesan and the pumpkin. Transfer the mixture to an ovenproof dish, sprinkle over the remaining mozzarella and two-thirds of the pecan crumb and cook for about 30 minutes or until bubbling and heated through. Serve with a green salad and the remaining pecan crumb on the side.

MIKE "THE SNAKE" NELSON'S STROMBOLI

SERVES 6–8
PREPARATION TIME: 1 HOUR, PLUS RISING
COOKING TIME: 1 HOUR 15 MINUTES

50g (generous ⅓ cup) pine nuts

125g (generous ½ cup) ricotta

3 dried figs, finely chopped

50g (½ cup) Pecorino or Parmesan cheese, finely chopped

125g (1¼ cups) mozzarella, finely chopped

1 tablespoon capers, rinsed and chopped

6 slices of prosciutto

12 slices of salami picante or chorizo

salt and pepper

Pizza dough

2½ teaspoons fast-action dried yeast or 15g (½oz) fresh yeast, crumbled

½ teaspoon salt

pinch of sugar

375g (2¾ cups) strong white flour, plus extra for dusting

200ml (scant 1 cup) warm water

2 tablespoons olive oil, plus extra for brushing

Tomato sauce

3 tablespoons olive oil

2 garlic cloves, sliced

leaves from 2 rosemary sprigs

500g (1lb 2oz) cherry tomatoes

❶ For the pizza dough, place the yeast, salt, sugar and flour in a large bowl. Gradually pour in the measured water and oil and, using a fork then your hands, form the mixture into a soft dough. Knead the dough on a lightly floured surface for 8–10 minutes until smooth and elastic, then place in a bowl, cover and leave in a warm place for about 1 hour or until doubled in size.

❷ For the sauce, place the oil in a saucepan over a medium heat and add the garlic and rosemary. When the garlic starts to colour, add the tomatoes, increase the heat, season and cover the pan. Cook, shaking the pan occasionally, for about 15 minutes or until the tomatoes are very tender. Press the tomato mixture through a fine sieve into a clean pan, pressing through as much of the flesh as possible. Place over a medium heat and bring to the boil. Reduce the heat and simmer for 10–15 minutes until thickened. Season to taste and leave to cool.

❸ Preheat the oven to 190°C (375°F), Gas Mark 5. Spread the pine nuts on a baking sheet and toast for 5–10 minutes until golden. Transfer to a plate to cool, then crush with a rolling pin. Place the ricotta in a bowl with the figs, Pecorino, mozzarella, capers and crushed pine nuts. Season and mix well. Set aside.

❹ Knead the dough briefly to knock all of the air out of it, then roll out on a lightly floured surface into a 45 x 35-cm (18 x 14-inch) rectangle. Spread the tomato sauce over the dough, leaving a 2-cm (¾-inch) border around the edge and lay the prosciutto in a single layer over the sauce. Spread evenly with the cheese mixture, dot with the salami and finally brush all round the edges with a little water.

❺ Tuck in the two short ends then roll up the stromboli to enclose the filling. Place it seam-side down on a large greased baking sheet and leave in a warm place for 30 minutes or until puffy. Increase the oven temperature to 220°C (425°F), Gas Mark 7. Brush the stromboli with oil, sprinkle with sea salt flakes and bake for 15 minutes on the bottom shelf of the oven. Reduce the heat to 200°C (400°F), Gas Mark 6 and bake for a further 25–30 minutes on the middle shelf until golden brown. Cut into slices to serve.

THE HORNE BROTHERS' BRIE & BUTTER BAGUETTES

SERVES 7
PREPARATION TIME: 1 HOUR, PLUS RESTING AND RISING
COOKING TIME: 25 MINUTES

1.05kg (7¾ cups) strong white flour, plus extra for dusting

2½ teaspoons fast-action dried yeast or 30g (1oz) fresh yeast, crumbled

3 teaspoons salt

about 700ml (3 cups) water

butter, for spreading

sliced Brie cheese, for filling

❶ Place the flour in a large bowl with the yeast and salt. Gradually add the water until the mixture just comes together and forms a sticky, rough dough. Wet your hands and scrape the dough on to a clean work surface using a plastic scraper or a fork. To knead, work quickly without adding extra flour. With a hand under each side, lift the dough and stretch it upwards, then slap it down away from you, folding it loosely over itself to trap air. Repeat in a continuous motion for 15 minutes until the dough becomes smooth and elastic and leaves the work surface more easily. It will be sticky to start with, but persevere and don't add more flour.

❷ Dust the dough with a little flour and form into a ball. Cover and rest in a warm place for 1 hour.

❸ Press out the dough on a lightly floured surface into a large square, then fold down the top third into the middle and press along the seam to seal. Turn by 180° and repeat. Divide the dough into 7 equal pieces. Taking one piece of dough at a time, repeat the pressing and folding (as above) and seal the dough pieces, then turn them over so the seams are underneath. You should now have 7 sausage shapes.

❹ Take one piece of dough and, starting from one end, fold one long side up and over to meet the other long side, twisting the dough as you go and pressing along the seam to seal. Keeping the seam underneath, squash the dough again and repeat this action once more, twisting and folding along its length. Now, using your flat palms, roll and stretch out the dough slightly to create its final baguette shape. Lay the shaped baguettes on a pleated floured tea towel and rest in a warm place for 1 hour.

❺ Preheat the oven to 230°C (450°F), Gas Mark 8. Place a roasting tin in the bottom of the oven and boil a full kettle of water. Arrange the baguettes on lightly floured baking sheets and sprinkle the tops with a little extra flour. Use a sharp blade or knife to cut a long slit down the length of each baguette. As you place the trays in the oven, pour boiling water into the roasting tin. Bake for 25 minutes or until evenly golden, then cool on a wire rack. They are best served the same day.

❻ Split the cooled baguettes lengthways, spread with butter and fill with sliced Brie.

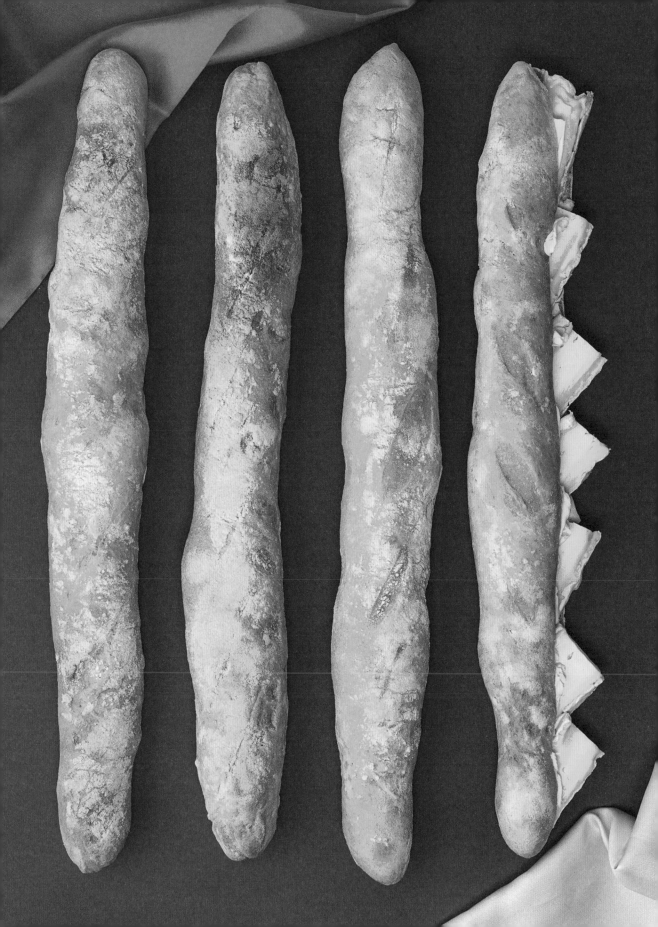

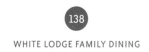
FAT TROUT TRAILER PARK'S
TROUT WITH CAPER BUTTER

SERVES 4
PREPARATION TIME: 15 MINUTES
COOKING TIME: 7–8 MINUTES

1 tablespoon wholegrain or Dijon mustard

4 large trout fillets with skin, about 200g (7oz) each

25g (2 tablespoons) unsalted butter

1 tablespoon olive oil

salt and pepper

boiled potatoes, to serve

Caper butter

2 lemons

25g (2 tablespoons) unsalted butter

1 tablespoon small capers, rinsed and chopped

1 tablespoon finely chopped tarragon

❶ Rub the mustard on the flesh sides of the trout fillets, season on both sides and set aside.

❷ For the caper butter, finely grate the zest from the lemons, then use a sharp knife to remove the skin and pith. Working over a bowl to catch the juices, cut the lemons into segments by cutting either side of the membrane and removing the flesh. Place the segments in the bowl and squeeze over any remaining juice from the pulp.

❸ To cook the trout, heat the butter with the oil in a large frying pan over a medium heat until foaming. Arrange the trout fillets in the pan, skin-side down, and cook for 3 minutes. Turn them over and cook for another 1–2 minutes or until just tender, then transfer to a serving platter and keep warm.

❹ For the caper butter, add the butter to the pan and heat gently until it starts to foam and turns light brown. It will smell sweet and nutty, but be careful not to burn it. Add the capers, lemon zest, lemon segments and tarragon. Heat through, then pour in the lemon juice and cook for 30 seconds. Season to taste, then pour over the trout on the platter and serve immediately with boiled potatoes.

THE WHITE LODGE DOPPELGÄNGER WHITE BEAN SALAD

SERVES 4
PREPARATION TIME: 30 MINUTES,
PLUS OVERNIGHT SOAKING
COOKING TIME: 1 HOUR 15 MINUTES

250g (2¼ cups) dried cannellini or haricot beans, soaked overnight in cold water

1 head of garlic, halved horizontally

1 fennel bulb, finely sliced

4 tablespoons extra virgin olive oil

juice of 1 lemon

1 teaspoon fennel seeds, crushed

1 green chilli, finely chopped

groundnut oil, for deep-frying

2 large white onions, thinly sliced into rings

3 tablespoons mint leaves, roughly torn or chopped

1 head of white chicory, leaves separated and roughly sliced

salt and pepper

❶ Drain and rinse the soaked beans, then place in a large saucepan with the garlic and cover with cold water. Bring to the boil, then reduce the heat and simmer, skimming away any scum that rises to the surface, for 45–60 minutes until tender.

❷ Place the fennel in a large bowl, drizzle with the olive oil and lemon juice and sprinkle with the crushed fennel seeds and chilli. Season, toss well and set aside.

❸ Heat the oil in a large, deep saucepan or deep-fat fryer to 180–190°C (350–375°F) or until a cube of bread browns in 30 seconds. Carefully lower the sliced onions, in batches, into the hot oil and cook until golden and crisp, taking care not to burn them. Drain on kitchen paper and set aside.

❹ Once the beans are tender, drain away the liquid and discard the garlic. Toss the beans with the fennel mixture, allow to cool a little, then stir in the mint and chicory. Taste and adjust the seasoning if necessary. Serve at room temperature, sprinkled with the fried onions.

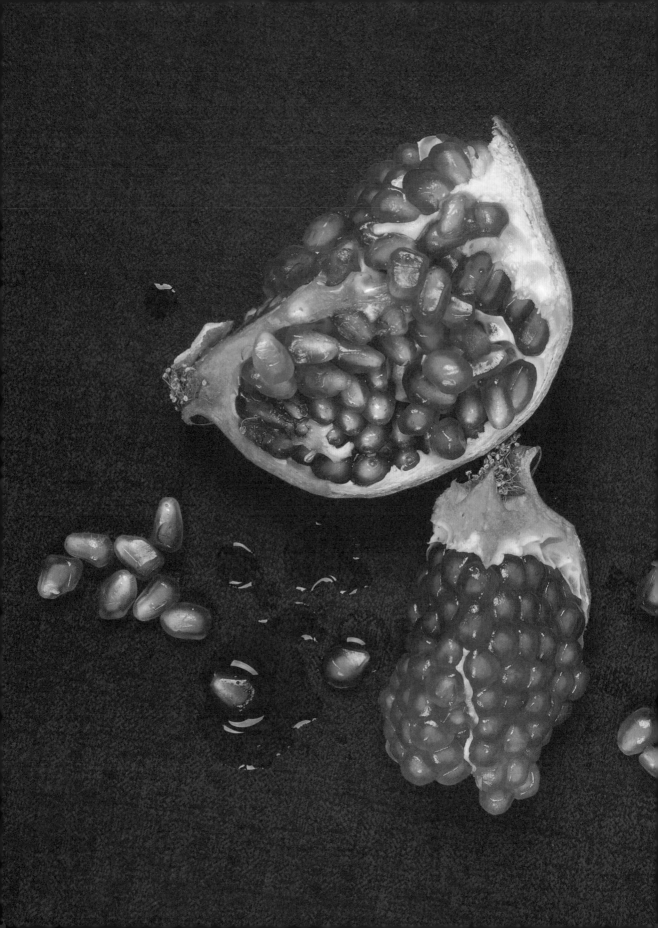

chapter 5

BLACK LODGE SUPPER CLUB

THE BLACK LODGE

In *Twin Peaks* any mention of the Black Lodge can turn your thoughts to darkness. It is the dwelling place of the spirits that inhabit the chosen few, where time hardly passes and all who visit hear the call of the owl and witness a flash of white light. It is said when Jupiter and Saturn meet, the door to the Black Lodge will be open and that fear will open that door.

Inside the Black Lodge dwell the doppelgangers, the shadow selves of each human in the physical world. When Agent Cooper visits the Black Lodge in the final episode of *Twin Peaks*, he comes face to face with his own doppelganger and has to fight to save his soul.

The repeating decor of the Black Lodge, the chevron floor with the red drapes, gives a striking impression of elegance and seductiveness but also hints at disorientation and unsettlement.

The recipes in this section are designed to bring you into the world of the desirable, the provocative and the beguiling. In short, into the world of the Black Lodge.

The chevron floor of the Black Lodge in Twin Peaks also appears in Lynch's first feature film *Eraserhead*. It is the lobby floor of Henry's house.

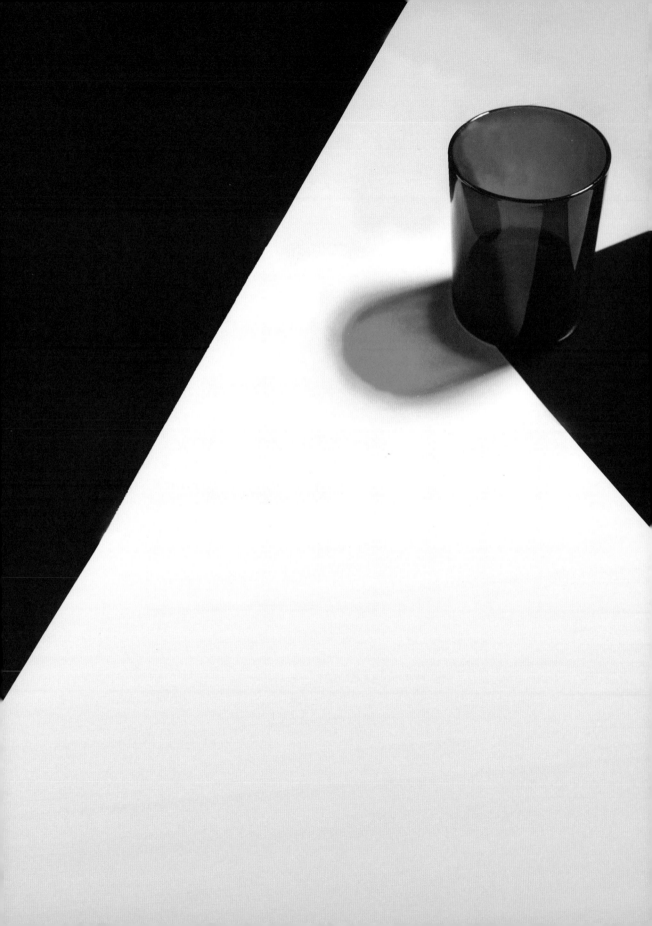

LELAND PALMER'S BUFFALO JOINT

SERVES 6–8
PREPARATION TIME: 1 HOUR 45 MINUTES
**COOKING TIME: 1 HOUR 15 MINUTES–
2 HOURS**

3kg (6lb 8oz) piece of buffalo or beef
rib on the bone

2 tablespoons olive oil

5 shallots, thickly sliced

a few thyme sprigs

450ml (scant 2 cups) red wine

450ml (scant 2 cups) port

salt and pepper

Braised red wine shallots

3 tablespoons olive oil

25g (2 tablespoons) butter

15 shallots or baby onions, peeled

a few thyme sprigs

2 teaspoons sugar

300ml (1¼ cups) red wine

200ml (scant 1 cup) chicken or beef stock

❶ Take the meat out of the refrigerator at least 1 hour before you plan to cook it. Preheat the oven to 220°C (425°F), Gas Mark 7. Massage the meat with the oil, then rub all over with salt and pepper. Sit the joint on a rack in a large roasting tin and cook for 15 minutes until browned all over.

❷ Reduce the heat to 150°C (300°F), Gas Mark 2. Calculate the remaining cooking time from this point, allowing 12 minutes per 500g (1lb 2oz) for rare, 15 minutes for medium, or 20 minutes for well done. Alternatively, test the joint with a meat thermometer; the temperature will reach 55°C (131°F) for rare, 60°C (140°F) for medium or 72°C (162°F) for well done. Turn the beef over halfway through cooking.

❸ Meanwhile, for the shallots, heat the oil and butter in a large frying pan over a medium heat, add the shallots and thyme, season and cook 5–10 minutes until lightly golden. Sprinkle over the sugar and cook for another 10 minutes, shaking the pan and turning the shallots occasionally so they colour evenly. Increase the heat, add the red wine and stock and cook until reduced by two-thirds.

❹ When the meat is ready, transfer it on its rack to a large plate and set aside to rest in a warm place for 15–20 minutes. Pour away the fat from the roasting tin and place the tin on the stove over a medium heat. Add the sliced shallots and thyme and cook for 5–6 minutes until softened. Add the red wine and port, then bubble over a high heat for 5 minutes.

❺ Use a slotted spoon to lift the whole shallots out of their cooking liquid and set aside in a warm place. Pour the cooking liquid into the roasting tin and simmer for 10–15 minutes or until reduced by half. Pour any juices from the resting meat into the sauce and season to taste. Carve the meat and serve with the shallots and sauce on the side.

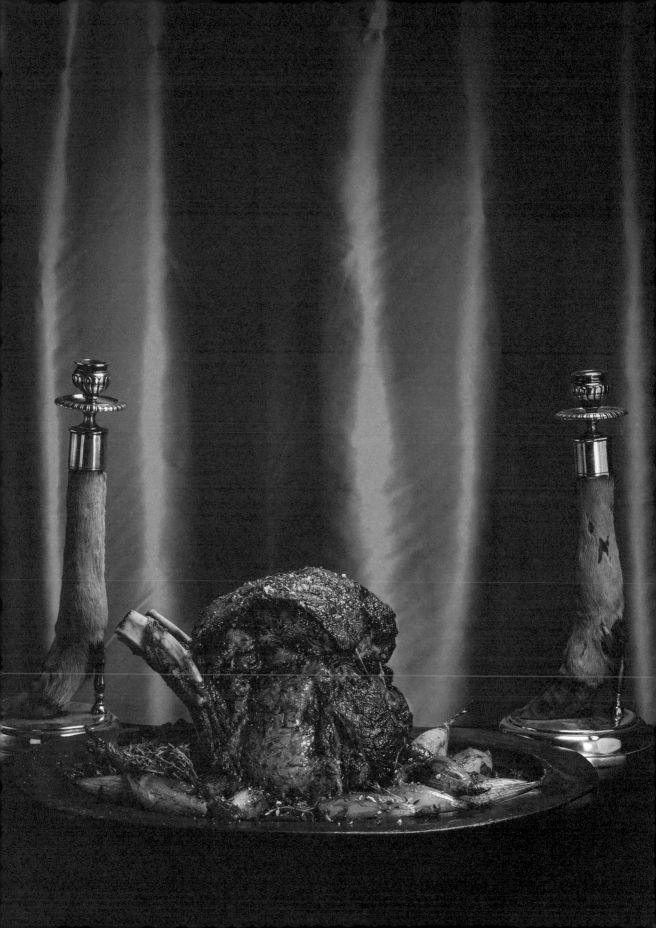

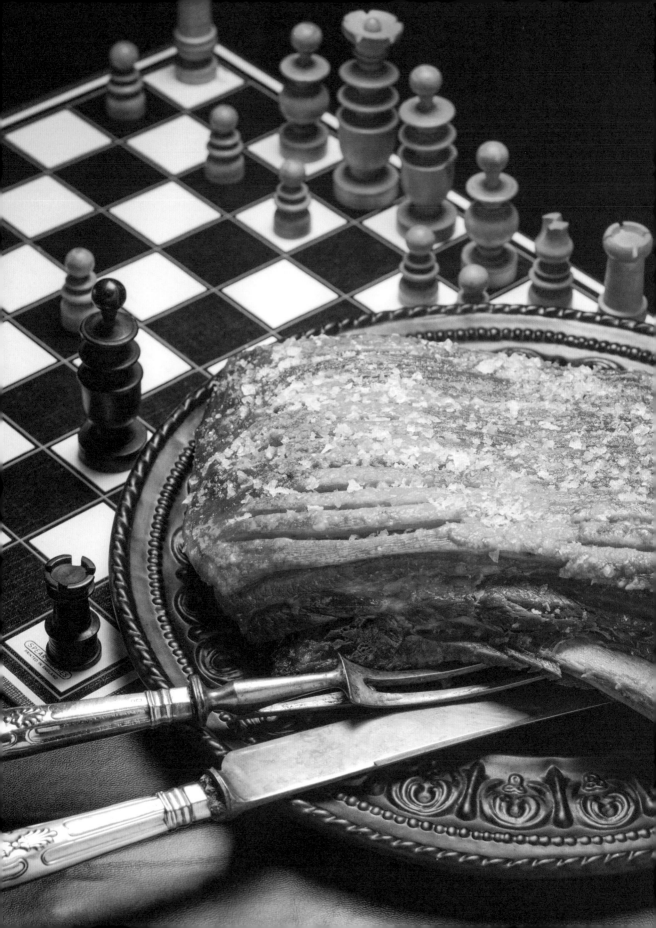

WINDOM EARLE'S BEER-MARINATED PORK BELLY

SERVES 6–8
PREPARATION TIME: 20 MINUTES
COOKING TIME: 6–7 HOURS, PLUS RESTING

2 dried chipotle chillies

1 dried ancho chilli

2 red onions, thickly sliced

2 tablespoons dark soft brown sugar

1 teaspoon fennel seeds

1 star anise

2 teaspoons smoked paprika

bunch of thyme

3 bay leaves

1 head of garlic, peeled

5-cm (2-inch) piece of fresh root ginger, peeled and chopped

1 tablespoon black peppercorns

1 cinnamon stick

2 apples, roughly chopped

600ml (2½ cups) dark beer

2kg (4lb 6oz) piece of pork belly on the bone

1 tablespoon apple cider vinegar

100g (⅔ cup) plain dark chocolate, chopped

sea salt flakes

❶ Place the chillies in a bowl and add boiling water to cover. Leave to soften for 15 minutes, then drain (keeping the liquid) and chop roughly. Preheat the oven to 220°C (425°F), Gas Mark 7.

❷ Place the onions in a large casserole or roasting tin with the sugar, fennel seeds, star anise, paprika, thyme, bay leaves, garlic, ginger, peppercorns, cinnamon, apples, beer and chilli-soaking liquid. Place over a high heat and bring to the boil.

❸ Rub the pork rind all over with sea salt flakes, then place the pork, skin-side up, in the casserole or tin on top of the other ingredients. Nestle the pork in but keep the skin above the level of the liquid. Cook in the oven for 30 minutes, then cover with foil or a lid, reduce the heat to 110°C (225°F), Gas Mark ¼ and cook for 6–7 hours, basting from time to time and topping up with water (or more beer) if necessary.

❹ Remove the foil, increase the heat to 220°C (425°F), Gas Mark 7 and cook for 30–40 minutes until the skin is crispy. Transfer the pork to a plate and leave it to rest in a warm place for at least 20 minutes.

❺ Strain the liquid into a clean saucepan over a high heat, pressing the vegetables with the back of a spoon to remove all the juices. Bring to the boil, then lower the heat and simmer until reduced by one-third. Season to taste, then stir in the vinegar and chocolate. Serve the sauce with the sliced pork.

The chess game corpse in the Sheriff's station was played by Kyle Maclachlan's brother Craig.

FILET MIGNON STUFFED WITH BLUE CHEESE

SERVES 4
PREPARATION TIME: 1 HOUR,
PLUS MARINATING
COOKING TIME: 45 MINUTES

6 tablespoons balsamic vinegar

4 tablespoons olive oil

2 garlic cloves, crushed

1 tablespoon wholegrain or Dijon mustard

leaves from 3–4 thyme sprigs

4 fillet steaks, 200–250g (7–9oz) each

4 slices of blue cheese

salt and pepper

Crispy bacon mash

250g (9oz) streaky bacon (about 10 rashers)

1kg (2lb 4oz) potatoes, peeled and cut into large chunks

50g (3½ tablespoons) butter

6 spring onions, finely chopped

100ml (scant ½ cup) milk

Griddled asparagus with pecan crumb

50g (3½ tablespoons) butter

400g (14oz) asparagus spears, trimmed and halved

50g (scant ½ cup) pecans, roughly crushed

25g (½ cup) fresh white breadcrumbs

finely grated zest of 1 lemon

❶ Place the balsamic vinegar, oil, garlic, mustard and thyme in a large shallow dish and whisk to combine. Make a small slit in the side of each steak and push in a piece of blue cheese. Place the steaks in the marinade and turn to coat. Cover and leave to marinate for 1–2 hours, turning once.

❷ For the mash, arrange the bacon on a large baking sheet. Place in a cold oven, set the temperature to 200°C (400°F), Gas Mark 6 and cook for 15–20 minutes or until crispy. Drain on kitchen paper until cool, then crumble into 2-cm (¾-inch) pieces. Cook the potatoes in a saucepan of water until tender. Drain, return to the pan and place back over a low heat for a few minutes to get rid of excess moisture, shaking to prevent burning.

❸ Melt the butter in a saucepan over a medium heat, add the spring onions and cook for 2–3 minutes until softened. Add the milk, season and cook for 2–3 minutes, then set aside.

❹ Place a large, heavy-based frying pan over a high heat. When very hot, cook the steaks for 15–20 seconds, then turn and cook for a further 15–20 seconds. Repeat for 2–3 minutes until browned on the outside yet pink in the middle. Transfer to a plate and leave to rest for 5 minutes.

❺ Pour the marinade into the hot pan, reduce the heat and simmer for 1–2 minutes or until thickened into a sauce.

❻ Mash the potatoes, stir in the milk and spring onion mixture, crumble in three-quarters of the crispy bacon and beat well.

❼ For the asparagus, melt the butter in a frying pan over a medium-high heat. Stir-fry the asparagus for 2 minutes. Add the pecans and cook for 2 minutes more until starting to toast, then add the breadcrumbs and continue cooking until the asparagus is tender and the pecans and breadcrumbs are toasted. Remove from the heat and stir in the lemon zest.

❽ Divide the mash between 4 plates and arrange the steaks on top. Drizzle with a little of the sauce, sprinkle with the remaining crispy bacon and serve with the asparagus.

THE GIANT'S SPECIAL GOOSE

SERVES 6
PREPARATION TIME: 45 MINUTES
COOKING TIME: 4–4½ HOURS

1 head of garlic

750g (1lb 10oz) sweet potatoes

850g (1lb 14oz) floury potatoes

50g (3½ tablespoons) butter

2 leeks, finely sliced

2 rosemary sprigs

1 tablespoon olive oil

450g (1lb) black pudding, roughly chopped

4.5kg (10lb) goose

125ml (½ cup) cider, dry sherry or marsala

400ml (1⅔ cups) chicken stock

salt and pepper

Baked apples

8 small eating apples

25g (2 tablespoons) butter

juice of 2 clementines or 1 large orange

1½ tablespoons light soft brown sugar

25g (scant ¼ cup) hazelnuts, crushed

2 heads of chicory, sliced into 2-cm (¾-inch) pieces

❶ Preheat the oven to 200°C (400°C), Gas Mark 6. Wrap the garlic in foil. Prick the potatoes and place on a baking sheet with the garlic. Bake for 1 hour until all the vegetables are tender, checking and removing the sweet potatoes after about 40 minutes. Leave to cool a little. Meanwhile, melt the butter in a saucepan over a medium–low heat, add the leeks and rosemary and cook for about 20 minutes until very soft.

❷ Peel the potatoes and sweet potatoes, tip the flesh into a bowl and mash. Squeeze the softened garlic flesh from its skins and mash into the potatoes with the leeks. Season well. Heat the oil in a nonstick frying pan over a high heat, add the black pudding and cook for 2 minutes, stirring occasionally, until it starts to change colour. Fold into the mash.

❸ Remove the 2 lumps of fat from inside the goose cavity. Prick the skin all over. Sprinkle salt into the cavity, then stuff it with the potato mixture and tie the legs with string. Rub with more salt, then place on a wire rack over a roasting tin. Roast for 40 minutes, then reduce the heat to 180°C (350°F), Gas Mark 4 and cook for 2–2½ hours more, pouring out fat from the tin now and then. To check for doneness, insert a skewer into the thickest part of the leg. If the juices run clear, the goose is ready. Transfer to a large plate, cover with foil and rest for 20–30 minutes.

❹ Meanwhile, prepare the apples. Score the skin in a horizontal band about one-third of the way from the top of each apple and arrange them in an ovenproof dish. Dot with the butter, drizzle with the orange juice, then sprinkle over the sugar and the hazelnuts. Cook in the oven for 1 hour or until tender, adding the chicory for the last 10 minutes of cooking.

❺ For the gravy, skim off as much fat from the roasting tin as possible. Place the tin over a medium heat, then add the cider, stirring with a wooden spoon to scrape up any bits stuck to the tin. Bring to the boil, lower the heat and simmer until reduced by half. Add the stock and boil again until slightly thickened.

❻ Present the goose on a platter, surrounded by the apples with their juices spooned over them, with gravy on the side.

R-B-T OPEN RAVIOLI WITH BLOODY MARY FILLING

SERVES 6 GENEROUSLY
PREPARATION TIME: 30 MINUTES
COOKING TIME: 3–3½ HOURS

2 tablespoons olive oil

250g (generous 1 cup) minced pork

250g (generous 1 cup) minced beef

1 garlic clove, finely chopped

1 large onion, finely chopped

1 large carrot, finely chopped

6 celery sticks, finely chopped

a few thyme sprigs

400ml (1⅔ cups) beef stock or water

18 squares of fresh lasagne, about 11 x 11cm (4¼ inches) each

50g (½ cup) Castelmagno or Parmesan cheese, finely grated

truffle oil, to drizzle

salt and pepper

Sauce

800g (4 cups) passata

4–6 tablespoons vodka

juice of 1 lemon

2 tablespoons Worcestershire sauce

½ teaspoon Tabasco sauce

1 tablespoon celery salt

1 teaspoon sugar

1 tablespoon horseradish sauce or 3cm (1¼ inches) fresh horseradish, finely grated

2 tablespoons olive oil

2 garlic cloves, thinly sliced

❶ Heat the oil in a large heavy-based saucepan over a high heat, add the minced meat in batches and cook, stirring occasionally, for about 20 minutes until golden. Add the garlic, onion, carrot, celery and thyme and cook, stirring, for a further 10 minutes.

❷ Place all the sauce ingredients, except the oil and garlic, in a large jug and stir to combine. Pour three-quarters of the sauce into the pan, add the stock and season well with pepper. Bring back to the boil, then reduce the heat and simmer for 2–2½ hours until the sauce is thick. Taste the sauce and add more celery salt, Tabasco, Worcestershire sauce, horseradish or pepper if necessary.

❸ Meanwhile, heat the remaining oil in a medium saucepan over a high heat, add the sliced garlic and just as it starts to colour, pour in the remaining tomato sauce. Bring to the boil, reduce the heat and simmer for about 20 minutes or until thickened. Season to taste.

❹ Cook the squares of pasta in a large saucepan of lightly salted boiling water until tender. Place a square of pasta on each plate, top with a large spoonful of the meat mixture and a sprinkling of the cheese. Add another layer of pasta, meat and cheese, then top with a final square of pasta. Spoon over the tomato sauce. Sprinkle with a little more cheese, drizzle with truffle oil and serve immediately.

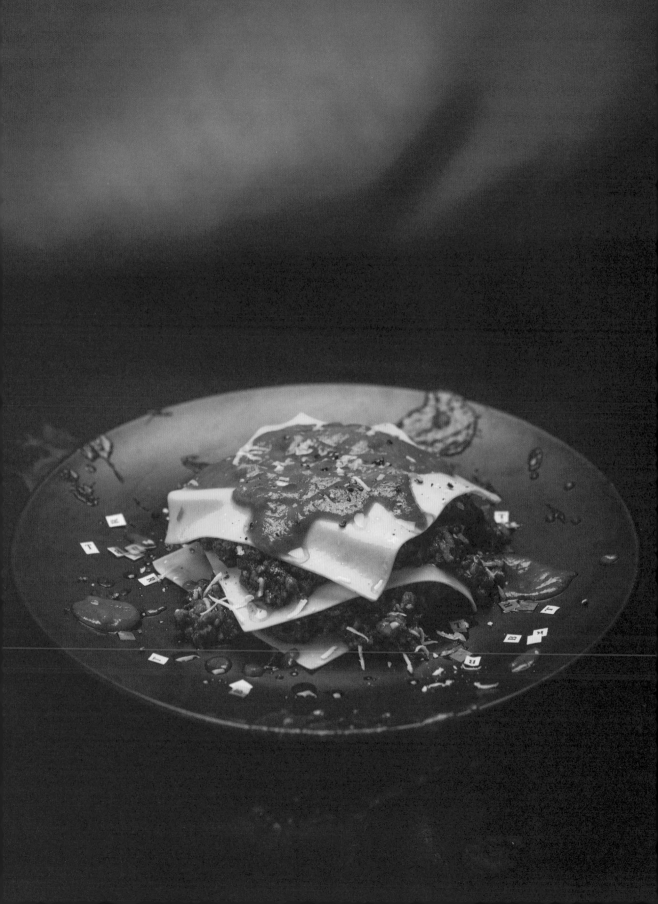

AGENT COOPER'S DUCKS ON THE LAKE

SERVES 6
PREPARATION TIME: 1 HOUR,
PLUS MARINATING
COOKING TIME: 3 HOURS 20 MINUTES
–3 HOURS 40 MINUTES

1 large duck, cut into 6–8 pieces

8 tablespoons sea salt

12 juniper berries, crushed

6 bay leaves, torn into pieces

a few thyme sprigs

pared rind from 1 large orange

about 750g (1lb 10oz) duck fat

salt and pepper

Potatoes

800g (1lb 12oz) potatoes

leaves from 6 rosemary sprigs

100ml (scant ½ cup) olive oil

1 head of garlic

Pear and pomegranate salad

juice of 1 lemon

1 teaspoon Dijon mustard

2 tablespoons olive oil

1 large ripe pear, cored and sliced

2 heads of chicory, leaves separated

1 small pomegranate

1 Place the duck pieces in a shallow non-metallic dish and rub the salt and crushed juniper berries evenly over them. Grind over some pepper, tuck in the bay leaves, thyme and strips of pared orange rind, then cover and marinate in the refrigerator for at least 6 hours or overnight.

2 Preheat the oven to 110°C (225°F), Gas Mark ¼. Brush the salt off the duck, reserving the herbs and orange rind.

3 Heat the duck fat in a heavy-based casserole in which the duck pieces will fit snugly. Bring the fat to a gentle simmer – it should just be quivering – then slide in the duck pieces. There should be enough fat to completely cover the duck. Bake for 2½–3 hours until soft and tender. Allow the duck to cool in the fat, then chill in the refrigerator until ready to use.

4 Preheat the oven to 220°C (425°F), Gas Mark 7. Slice the potatoes very thinly, leaving the skins on, then divide between 2 large baking sheets. Scatter with the rosemary, drizzle with the oil and season well with salt and pepper. Break the garlic bulb apart and scatter a few whole, unpeeled cloves over each sheet. Mix everything together with your hands and spread out in a single layer.

5 Place the sheets on the top and middle shelves of the oven and cook for 40–50 minutes, turning the potatoes occasionally and swapping the sheet positions halfway through cooking.

6 Scrape most of the fat from the duck pieces, then arrange on top of the potatoes for the last 20 minutes of cooking, and cook until the duck skin is crisp.

7 Meanwhile, make the salad. Place the lemon juice, mustard and olive oil in a salad bowl, season and whisk to combine. Add the pear and chicory and toss to coat. Cut the pomegranate into quarters and remove the skin and all the bitter pith. Add the seeds to the salad and toss well.

8 Serve the duck on top of the salad.

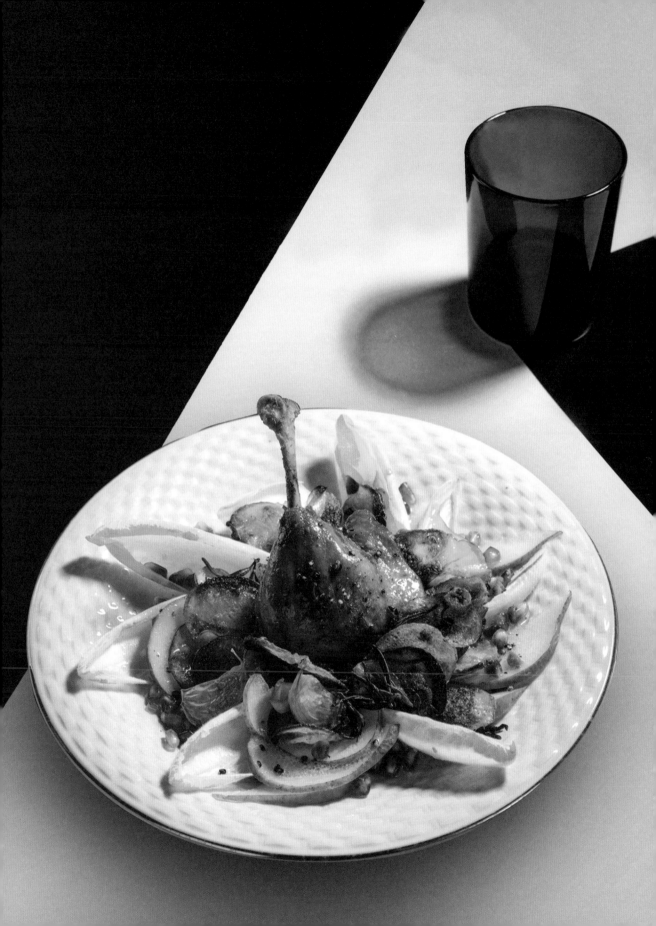

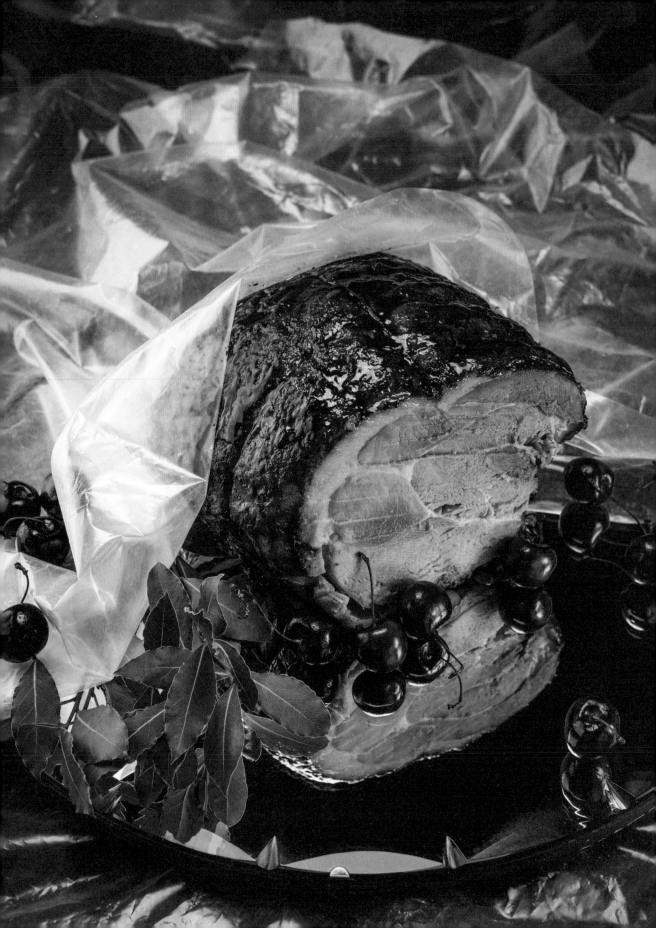

MADDY FERGUSON'S CHERRY COLA HAM

SERVES 15–20
PREPARATION TIME: 20 MINUTES, PLUS
HOMEMADE CHERRY COLA RECIPE TIME,
IF USING
COOKING TIME: 3 HOURS 45 MINUTES

3kg (6lb 8oz) uncooked boneless ham joint

1 quantity Homemade Cherry Cola (see page 70) with all the flavouring ingredients left in, or 3 litres (2¾ quarts) shop-bought cherry cola

3 onions, quartered

4 bay leaves, plus extra to garnish

4 tablespoons molasses

4 tablespoons Dijon mustard

100ml (scant ½ cup) bourbon whiskey (optional)

fresh cherries, to garnish

❶ Place the ham in a large saucepan with the cherry cola. If using homemade cola, top up with 3 litres (2¾ quarts) of water. Add the onions and bay leaves, cover the pan and bring to the boil. Reduce the heat and simmer for about 3 hours, allowing 30 minutes per 500g (1lb 2oz) of ham.

❷ Remove the ham from the cooking liquid and preheat the oven to 160°C (325°F), Gas Mark 3. Slice the rind off the ham, leaving the underlying fat intact. Use a sharp knife to score the fat in a diamond pattern. Place the ham in a foil-lined roasting tin.

❸ Place the molasses, mustard and bourbon, if using, in a small bowl and mix well. Spread one-third of the mixture over the ham to glaze. Bake for 15 minutes, spread with another third of the glaze and return to the oven for another 15 minutes. Spread the remaining glaze over the ham and bake for a final 15 minutes.

❹ Allow to cool completely before slicing and serving garnished with fresh cherries and bay leaves.

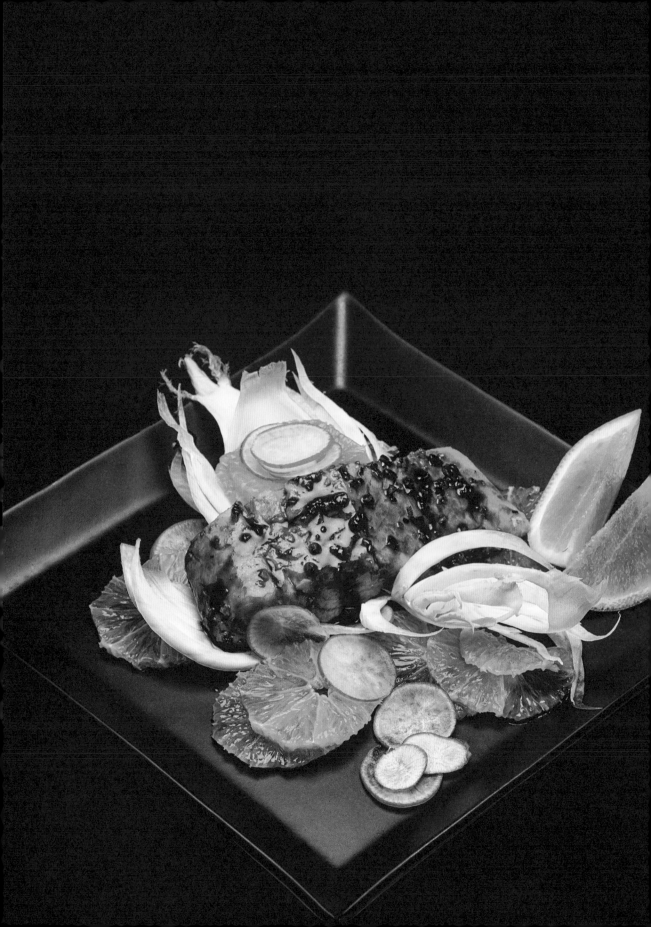

FIRE WALK HOT TEA SMOKED SALMON WITH BLOOD ORANGE, FENNEL & RADISH SALAD

SERVES 6
PREPARATION TIME: 30 MINUTES, PLUS MARINATING
COOKING TIME: 15 MINUTES

6 salmon fillets, about 150g (5½oz) each, with skin on

100g (½ cup) dark muscovado sugar

100g (½ cup) uncooked rice

100g (1¼ cups) tea leaves

salt and pepper

Marinade

1 garlic clove, crushed

100ml (scant ½ cup) strong espresso coffee

1 tablespoon dark muscovado sugar

1 tablespoon dark soy sauce

2 tablespoons black rice or balsamic vinegar

1 tablespoon sesame oil

2 tablespoons mirin

1 red chilli, finely chopped

Salad

6 blood oranges

2 tablespoons extra-virgin olive oil

2 heads of fennel, very finely sliced

8 radishes, very finely sliced

❶ Place all the marinade ingredients in a shallow dish and mix well. Add the salmon fillets, turn to coat and leave to marinate for 1 hour.

❷ Place the sugar, rice and tea leaves in a bowl and mix well. Line a wok or deep roasting tin with a double layer of foil, then place the tea mixture in the bottom. Place a trivet or wire rack over the top.

❸ Remove the salmon from the marinade, season and lay each piece on a small square of parchment paper. Arrange on the trivet and cover very tightly with a lid or a tent of foil. Place the wok or roasting tin over a medium heat for about 2 minutes until the tea just starts to smoulder.

❹ Reduce the heat to low and leave to smoke gently for 5 minutes. Remove from the heat and leave for a further 5 minutes, then remove the lid.

❺ Meanwhile, make the salad. Cut a thin slice from the top and bottom of 4 of the oranges. Working with one orange at a time, place it upright on a board and, using a sharp knife, slice strips from the orange from top to bottom to remove the peel and the pith. Rotate the orange and repeat until peeled. Cut the remaining oranges into slim wedges.

❻ Working over a bowl, cut between the membrane to remove the segments from the peeled oranges and drop into the bowl. Pour the olive oil into the bowl and season. Tip in the sliced fennel and radishes, season to taste and toss all together well.

❼ Pour the marinade into a small saucepan over a medium heat and bring to the boil. Reduce the heat and simmer for 3–4 minutes until thickened.

❽ Drizzle the sauce over the salmon and serve the salmon on a bed of the salad with extra wedges of orange on the side.

GARMONBOZIA CREAMED CORN

SERVES 4 AS A SIDE
PREPARATION TIME: 15 MINUTES
COOKING TIME: 20–25 MINUTES

4 sweetcorn cobs, husks and silks removed
25g (2 tablespoons) butter
1 small onion, finely chopped
200ml (scant 1 cup) water
300ml (1¼ cups) double cream
salt and pepper

❶ Use a large, sharp knife to trim the tops and bottoms from the sweetcorn cobs. One at a time, stand them on their bases and cut the kernels off the cobs from top to bottom, turning as you go. Then, with the point of a spoon, scrape down the cobs to remove any pulp.

❷ Melt the butter in a saucepan over a medium heat. Add the onion and cook gently for 5–6 minutes, without colouring, until softened.

❸ Add the corn kernels and pulp and measured water and bring to the boil. Reduce the heat, cover and simmer for 8–10 minutes or until the corn is tender.

❹ Add the cream, season to taste and bring back to the boil. Reduce the heat and simmer, uncovered, for 4–6 minutes until the mixture has thickened. Serve immediately.

Garmonbozia (definition) Pain manifested in the form of creamed corn.

TURKEY & AVOCADO SALAD

SERVES 4
PREPARATION TIME: 20 MINUTES

375g (13oz) cooked turkey

1 large avocado

punnet of mustard and cress

150g (5½oz) mixed salad leaves

50g (1¾oz) mixed toasted seeds, such as pumpkin and sunflower

Dressing

2 tablespoons apple juice

2 tablespoons natural yogurt

1 teaspoon clear honey

1 teaspoon wholegrain mustard

salt and pepper

1 Thinly slice the turkey. Peel, stone and dice the avocado and mix it with the mustard and cress and salad leaves in a large bowl. Add the turkey and toasted seeds and stir to combine.

2 Make the dressing by whisking together the apple juice, yogurt, honey and mustard. Season to taste with salt and pepper.

3 Pour the dressing over the salad and toss to coat. Serve the salad with toasted wholegrain rye bread or rolled up in flat breads.

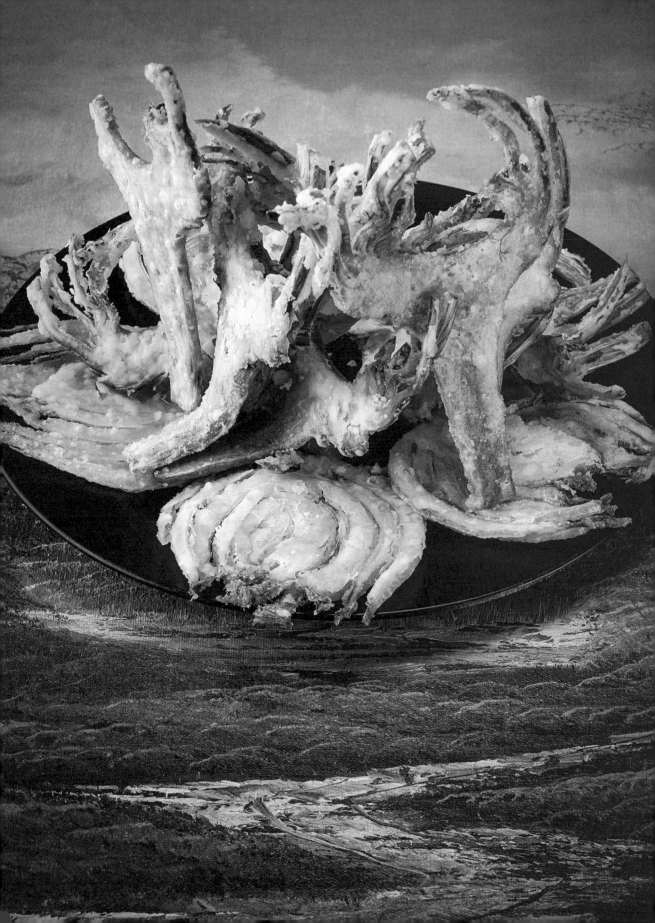

CIRCLE OF TREES

SERVES 6–8 AS A STARTER
PREPARATION TIME: 30 MINUTES
COOKING TIME: 20 MINUTES

2 fennel bulbs
8–12 small young globe artichokes
juice of 1 lemon
potato or rice flour, for dusting
groundnut oil, for deep-frying
sea salt flakes

1 Slice the fennel bulbs lengthways as thinly as possible (a mandolin would be good for this).

2 Remove the hard outer leaves from the artichokes, peel the tough stalks and trim them down to about 7cm (2¾ inches).

3 Use a serrated knife to cut about 3cm (1¼ inches) off the pointed tops of the artichokes, then use a spoon in a circular motion to scoop out the hairy chokes from the centres. Rub all the cut surfaces with lemon juice to prevent discolouration.

4 Cut the artichokes into fine slices lengthways from top to stalk (they'll look like little trees) and toss the sliced artichokes and fennel in potato flour to coat.

5 Heat the oil in a large, deep saucepan or deep-fat fryer to 180–190°C (350–375°F) or until a cube of bread browns in 30 seconds. Carefully lower the sliced artichokes, in batches, into the hot oil and cook for 3–4 minutes until golden and crisp. Drain on kitchen paper and toss with sea salt.

THE BLACK LODGE DOPPELGÄNGER BLACK BEAN SALAD

SERVES 4
PREPARATION TIME: 30 MINUTES, PLUS OVERNIGHT SOAKING
COOKING TIME: 4–5 HOURS

6 ripe tomatoes, halved

2 garlic cloves, finely chopped

4 tablespoons extra virgin olive oil

250g (1¼ cups) dried black beans, soaked overnight in cold water

2 tablespoons roughly torn or chopped basil leaves

salt and pepper

Dressing

2 tablespoons balsamic vinegar

2 tablespoons extra virgin olive oil

50g (⅓ cup) black olives, pitted and chopped

4 spring onions, finely chopped

1 red chilli, deseeded and finely chopped

2 tablespoons lemon or lime juice

1 Preheat the oven to 150°C (300°F), Gas Mark 2. Arrange the tomato halves, cut-sides up, on a baking sheet. Mix the garlic with the olive oil, season to taste and spoon or brush over the tomatoes.

2 Cook for 3–4 hours until tender, slightly shrunken but still bright red. If they become too dark they will taste bitter. Transfer to a plate and allow to cool.

3 For the dressing, scrape any tomato juices from the baking sheet into a large bowl and stir in the balsamic vinegar, olive oil, olives, spring onions, chilli and lemon or lime juice.

4 Drain and rinse the soaked beans, then place in a large saucepan and cover with cold water. Bring to the boil, then reduce the heat and simmer, skimming away any scum that rises to the surface, for 45–60 minutes until tender.

5 Once the beans are tender, drain away the liquid. Toss the beans with the dressing, allow to cool a little, then stir in the basil. Taste and adjust the seasoning if necessary. Serve at room temperature, topped with the roast tomatoes.

AGENT COOPER'S ASPARAGUS & ROCKET SALAD

SERVES 4
PREPARATION TIME: 15 MINUTES
COOKING TIME: ABOUT 5 MINUTES

3 tablespoons olive oil

500g (1lb 2oz) asparagus

125g (4½oz) rocket leaves

2 spring onions, finely sliced

4 radishes, finely sliced

salt and pepper

Tarragon and lemon dressing

finely grated rind of 2 lemons

4 tablespoons tarragon vinegar

2 tablespoons chopped tarragon

½ teaspoon Dijon mustard

pinch of caster sugar

150ml (⅔ cup) olive oil

To garnish

herbs, such as tarragon, parsley, chervil
and dill, roughly chopped

thin strips of lemon rind

❶ For the dressing, place the lemon rind, vinegar, tarragon, mustard and sugar in a small bowl and add salt and pepper to taste. Stir to mix, then gradually whisk in the oil. Alternatively, place all the ingredients in a screw-top jar with a lid and shake well to combine.

❷ Heat the oil in a large, nonstick frying pan and add the asparagus in a single layer. Cook for about 5 minutes, turning occasionally, until patched with brown and tender when pierced with the tip of a sharp knife. Remove from the pan to a shallow dish and sprinkle with salt and pepper. Cover with the dressing, toss gently and leave to stand for 5 minutes.

❸ Arrange the rocket on a serving plate and sprinkle the spring onions and radishes on top. Arrange the asparagus in a pile in the centre of the plate and garnish with herbs and lemon rind.

The strange way the characters talk in the Black Lodge was achieved by getting the actors to speak their lines backwards, then reversing the sound so they were being said the correct way.

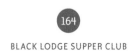
GHOSTWOOD GÂTEAU

Winner of a social-media competition to supply a recipe to appear in this cookbook. Congratulations, Hannah!

SERVES 12
**PREPARATION TIME: 1 HOUR 10 MINUTES,
PLUS COOLING AND FREEZING**
COOKING TIME: 40 MINUTES

100g (generous ½ cup) plain dark chocolate (minimum 70% cocoa solids), broken into cubes

175g (1½ sticks) lightly salted butter, plus extra for greasing

300g (scant 2½ cups) plain flour

375g (scant 2 cups) caster sugar

25g (¼ cup) cocoa powder

1 teaspoon bicarbonate of soda

pinch of salt

2 eggs

200ml (scant 1 cup) natural yogurt

100ml (scant ½ cup) boiling water

Filling and decorating

425g (15oz) can pitted cherries

4 tablespoons kirsch

125g (generous ⅓ cup) cherry jam

300ml (1¼ cups) double cream

4 tablespoons icing sugar

200g (generous 1 cup) plain dark chocolate (minimum 70% cocoa solids), broken into cubes

large handful of fresh cherries, to decorate

Ganache

200ml (scant 1 cup) double cream

250g (generous 1¼ cups) plain dark chocolate (minimum 70% cocoa solids), broken into cubes

1 Preheat the oven to 180°C (350°F), Gas Mark 4 and grease and line the bases of 3 cake tins, 20cm (8 inches) in diameter. Melt the chocolate and butter in a heatproof bowl set over a saucepan of gently simmering water, making sure the water does not touch the bottom of the bowl.

2 Place the flour in a large bowl with the caster sugar, cocoa powder, bicarbonate of soda and salt. Mix the eggs and yogurt in another bowl. Add the chocolate and egg mixtures to the dry ingredients with the measured water and mix with a hand-held electric whisk until smooth. Divide evenly between the prepared tins and level the surface. Bake for 25 minutes, swapping the positions of the tins after 20 minutes to ensure even cooking. The cakes are ready when a skewer inserted into the centre comes out clean. Leave to cool in their tins for 5 minutes.

3 Drain the canned cherries, reserving the juice. Mix 3 tablespoons of the juice with the kirsch. Turn the cakes out of their tins on to wire racks, then prick the surfaces with a skewer. Drizzle the kirsch mixture over and leave to cool. Mix the drained canned cherries and jam in a small bowl.

4 For the ganache, place the cream in a heavy-based saucepan over a low heat. Bring just to a simmer, then remove from the heat and add the chocolate. Stir until smooth, then set aside until spreadable. When the cakes are cool, whip the remaining cream with the icing sugar until soft peaks form. Spread over the tops of 2 of the cakes, then spoon the cherries on top. Place one of the topped cakes on a serving plate and arrange the other on top. Top with the plain cake, then spread the chocolate ganache evenly all over the cake to cover.

5 Melt the remaining chocolate in a heatproof bowl set over a saucepan of gently simmering water. Line 2 baking sheets with baking parchment and, using a piping bag fitted with a fine nozzle, pipe chocolate tree shapes on the paper. Place in the freezer for 5–10 minutes until the chocolate has hardened, then peel the trees off the paper and stick to the cake.

6 Pile the fresh cherries on and around the cake and serve.

A MANICURE INSPIRED BY TWIN PEAKS

This is based on an original concept by The Double R Club (*see* page 212).

You will need

Printer

Paper

Scissors

Clear nail polish

Tweezers

The method

1 Print the letters R, O, B and T on to printer paper in font size 10.

2 Cut out the letters into squares.

3 Paint one coat of clear nail polish on to the ring finger of the left hand and allow to dry until slightly tacky.

4 Using the tweezers, stick a single letter on to the clear nail polish and press down gently with the tweezers.

5 Paint a second coat of clear nail polish over the letter and allow to dry.

Fun fingernail facts – contains spoilers!

- Special Agent Dale Cooper concluded that these letters, placed under the fingernails of BOB's murder victims, would eventually spell out the name ROBERTSON.

- In *Fire Walk With Me,* Agent Sam Stanley discovers the letter T under the fingernail of Teresa Banks.

- Despite surviving BOB, Cooper found that Ronette Pulaski had the letter B under her fingernail.

- Of course the most famous of BOB's victims, Laura Palmer, had the letter R under her fingernail; her cousin Maddy Ferguson had the letter O.

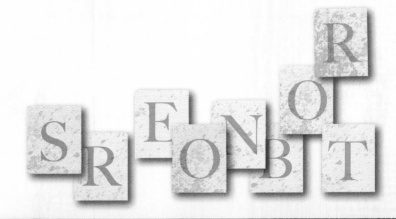

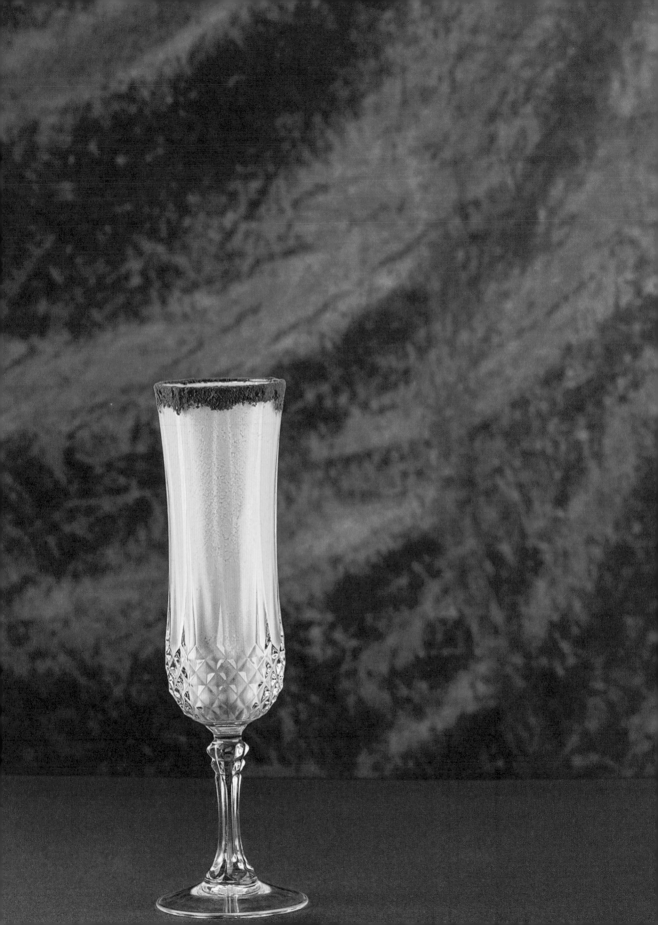

chapter 6

DESSERTS & COCKTAILS

DESSERTS & COCKTAILS

And now we come to my favourite section in the book. Here I had the opportunity to combine two of my favourite things: *Twin Peaks* and desserts. Pinch me! Everyone has a favourite dessert, although personally I would find it difficult to choose just one. Hopefully you will find a tempting variation of your favourite here.

Of course one key recipe inspired by *Twin Peaks* is the mighty Cherry Pie.

The RR Diner is famous for its Cherry Pie with Shelly proudly declaring that it is the best in the tri-counties. But this section offers a variety of pies to bake up, including a Vegan Cherry Pie.

When we think of desserts, we think of comfort or decadence, and the following recipes provide both of those. I wanted to give you desserts for entertaining, desserts for family dining and desserts for those moments when nothing else will do! And what better way to follow a mouth-watering dessert than with a luxurious cocktail? So tuck in and indulge in some damn fine after-dinner decadence!

Kyle MacLachlan doesn't like cherry pie! So during the filming of *Twin Peaks* he is actually eating berry pie.

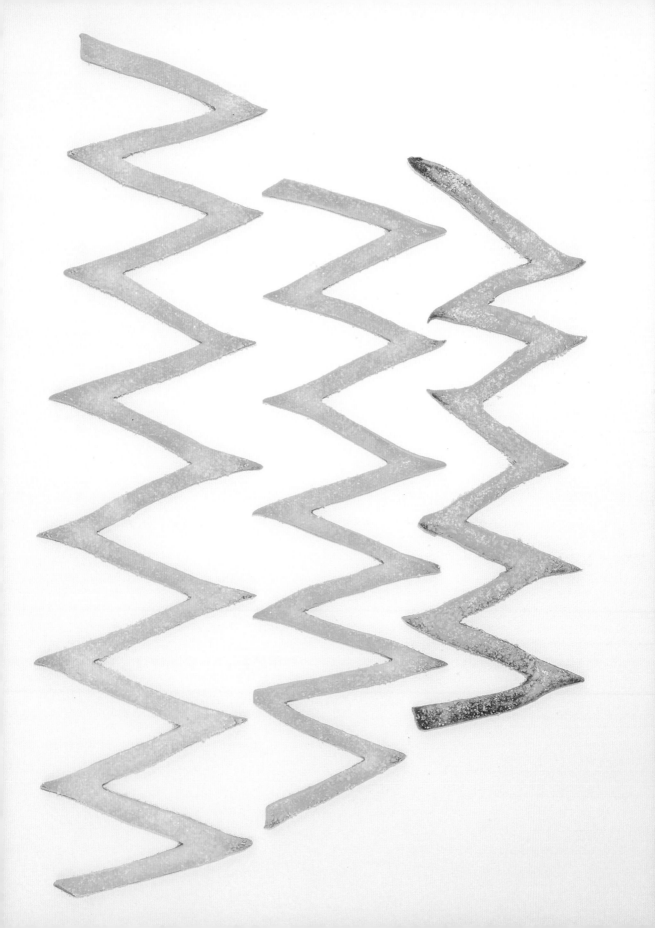

SHELLY JOHNSON'S CHERRY PIE

SERVES 8
PREPARATION TIME: 1 HOUR,
PLUS RESTING
COOKING TIME: ABOUT 1 HOUR

150g (generous ½ cup) cherry jam

150g (¾ cup) caster sugar

1½ tablespoons cornflour

3 tablespoons water or bourbon whiskey

1.25kg (2lb 12oz) sweet cherries, pitted
(750g/1lb 10oz pitted weight)

1 large egg yolk mixed with 1 tablespoon
water, for glazing

1 tablespoon granulated sugar

Pastry

450g (3⅔ cups) plain flour, plus extra
for dusting

50g (scant ½ cup) ground almonds

100g (generous ¾ cup) icing sugar

pinch of sea salt

250g (1¼ sticks) unsalted butter, cubed,
plus extra for greasing

1 large egg

½ teaspoon vanilla extract

5 tablespoons water

"When Norma isn't slaving away in the back of the RR Diner baking her famous pies, Shelly has been known to sneak back there with a glass of bourbon and try her hand at cherry pie. Enjoy!"

CAST MEMBER, MADCHEN AMICK

❶ For the pastry, place the flour, ground almonds, icing sugar and salt in a large mixing bowl and stir to combine. Add the butter and rub in with the fingertips until the mixture resembles fine breadcrumbs.

❷ Beat the egg with the vanilla extract and measured water. Stir the liquid into the flour with a fork, then your fingers, and bring the mixture together to form a firm dough. Divide the dough in half, flatten each portion into a disc, wrap in clingfilm and chill in the refrigerator for at least 1 hour.

❸ Meanwhile, place the jam and sugar in a saucepan over a medium heat and stir until the sugar has dissolved. Bring to the boil, then mix the cornflour and measured water or Bourbon together and stir into the cherry mixture. Bring to the boil again, stirring all the time, until thickened. Remove from the heat, add the cherries, mix well and leave to cool completely.

❹ Preheat the oven to 200°C (400°F), Gas Mark 6. Roll out one pastry disc on a lightly floured surface and use to line the base and sides of a greased 24-cm (9½-inch) pie dish (metal is best). Fill with the cherry mixture and brush the top of the pie edge with a little of the egg glaze.

❺ Thinly roll out the remaining pastry disc and cut into long zig-zag shapes. Arrange them on top of the pie, pressing to stick them to the pie base around the edges.

❻ Brush the pastry with more of the egg glaze and sprinkle over the sugar. Bake for about 20 minutes until the crust is golden, then reduce the temperature to 180°C (350°F), Gas Mark 4 and bake for a further 35–40 minutes until the filling is bubbling and the pastry is crisp, covering the pastry with foil, if necessary, to prevent it burning. Allow the pie to cool for about 1 hour before serving.

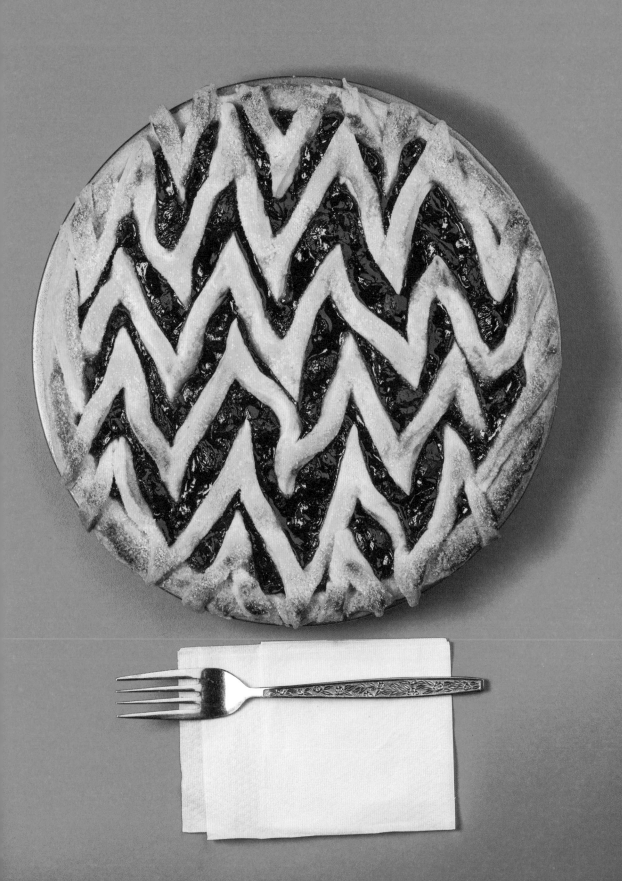

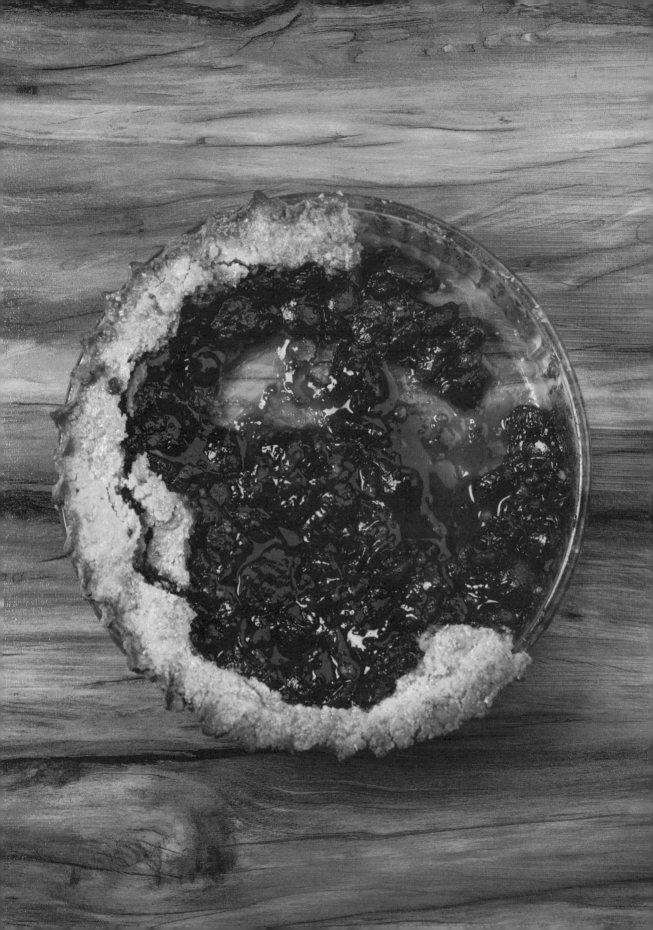

NORMA JENNINGS' VEGAN CHERRY PIE

SERVES 8
PREPARATION TIME: 1 HOUR,
PLUS RESTING
COOKING TIME: ABOUT 1 HOUR

150g (generous ½ cup) cherry jam

150g (¾ cup) caster sugar

1½ tablespoons cornflour

3 tablespoons cold water

1.25kg (2lb 12oz) sweet cherries, pitted
(750g/1lb 10oz pitted weight)

1 tablespoon demerara sugar

black coffee, to serve

Vegan pastry

250g (2 cups) plain flour, plus extra
for dusting

100g (½ cup) light muscovado sugar

75g (scant ¾ cup) ground almonds

pinch of salt

100g (7 tablespoons) coconut oil,
plus extra for greasing

½ teaspoon vanilla extract

4 tablespoons water

❶ For the pastry, place the flour, sugar, ground almonds and salt in a large mixing bowl and stir to combine. Add the coconut oil and rub in with the fingertips until the mixture resembles fine breadcrumbs.

❷ Mix the vanilla extract with the measured water. Stir the liquid into the flour with a fork, then your fingers, and bring the mixture together to form a soft dough. Divide the dough in half, flatten each portion into a disc, wrap in clingfilm and chill in the refrigerator for at least 1 hour.

❸ Meanwhile, place the jam and sugar in a saucepan over a medium heat and stir until the sugar has dissolved. Bring to the boil, then mix the cornflour and measured water together and stir into the cherry mixture. Bring to the boil again, stirring all the time, until thickened. Remove from the heat, add the cherries, mix well and leave to cool completely.

❹ Preheat the oven to 200°C (400°F), Gas Mark 6. Roll out one pastry disc on a lightly floured surface and use to line the base and sides of a greased 24-cm (9½-inch) pie dish (metal is best). Fill with the cherry mixture and brush the top of the pie edge with a little water.

❺ Thinly roll out the remaining pastry disc and lay on top of the pie, pressing and crimping the edges together to seal. Cut two small holes in the top of the pie to let out steam.

❻ Brush the pastry with water and sprinkle over the sugar. Bake for about 20 minutes until the crust is golden, then reduce the temperature to 180°C (350°F), Gas Mark 4 and bake for a further 35–40 minutes until the filling is bubbling and the pastry is crisp, covering the pastry with foil, if necessary, to prevent it burning. Allow the pie to cool for about 1 hour before serving with hot black coffee.

PEAR & ALMOND TART

SERVES 8
PREPARATION TIME: 20 MINUTES,
PLUS CHILLING
COOKING TIME: 50–55 MINUTES

1 quantity Sweet Shortcrust Pastry
(see page 181), chilled

flour, for dusting

125g (1⅛ sticks) unsalted butter, at room
temperature, plus extra for greasing

125g (generous ½ cup) caster sugar

125g (generous 1 cup) ground almonds

2 eggs, lightly beaten

1 tablespoon lemon juice

3 ripe pears, peeled, cored and thickly sliced

25g (generous ¼ cup) flaked almonds

icing sugar, for dusting

vanilla ice cream, to serve

Chocolate sauce

100g (scant ⅔ cup) plain dark chocolate
(minimum 70% cocoa solids), chopped

50g (3½ tablespoons) unsalted butter, diced

1 tablespoon golden syrup

❶ Roll out the pastry on a lightly floured surface and
use to line a greased 24-cm (9½-inch) tart tin. Trim off the
excess with scissors so it stands just above the top of the tin.
Prick the base with a fork, then chill in the refrigerator for
30 minutes. Preheat the oven to 190°C (375°F), Gas Mark 5.

❷ Line the pastry case with baking parchment and part-fill
with baking beans. Bake blind for 15 minutes or until lightly
golden, then remove the paper and beans and cook for a
further 5–10 minutes. Leave to cool completely. Reduce the
oven temperature to 180°C (350°F), Gas Mark 4.

❸ Beat the butter, sugar and ground almonds together
until smooth, then beat in the eggs and lemon juice.

❹ Arrange the pear slices in the pastry case and carefully
spread over the almond mixture. Sprinkle with the flaked
almonds and bake for 30 minutes until the topping is golden
and firm to the touch. Leave to cool.

❺ For the chocolate sauce, place all the ingredients in
a saucepan over a gentle heat and stir until melted and
smooth. Leave to cool slightly.

❻ Dust the tart with icing sugar and serve in wedges with
the chocolate sauce and some vanilla ice cream.

MAJOR BRIGGS'S HUCKLEBERRY PIE

SERVES 6–8
PREPARATION TIME: 40 MINUTES,
PLUS CHILLING
COOKING TIME: 1–1½ HOURS

150g (scant ¾ cup) brown sugar

75g (scant ¾ cup) ground almonds

2 tablespoons plain flour

pinch of ground nutmeg

500g (5 cups) huckleberries or blueberries, defrosted and drained if frozen

1 tablespoon lemon juice

pinch of salt

1 tablespoon granulated sugar

Pastry

350g (generous 2¾ cups) plain flour, plus extra for dusting

100g (generous ¾ cup) icing sugar

pinch of salt

180g (1⅝ sticks) butter, cubed, plus extra for greasing

180g (generous ¾ cup) cream cheese

½ teaspoon vanilla extract

❶ For the pastry, place the flour, icing sugar and salt in a large mixing bowl and stir to combine. Add the butter and rub in with the fingertips until the mixture resembles fine breadcrumbs.

❷ Add the cream cheese and vanilla and rub into the mixture until evenly blended to form a soft dough. Flatten into a disc, wrap in cling film and chill in the refrigerator for at least 1 hour.

❸ Mix the brown sugar, almonds, flour and nutmeg together. Add huckleberries, lemon juice and salt and toss together.

❹ Preheat the oven to 200°C (400°F), Gas Mark 6. Roll out two-thirds of the pastry on a lightly floured surface and use to line the base of a greased 22–24-cm (8½–9½-inch) pie plate. Fill with the huckleberry mixture and brush the top of the pie edge with a little water.

❺ Thinly roll out the remaining pastry and lay on top of the pie, pressing and crimping the edges together to seal. Reroll any trimmings and use to cut out shapes to decorate the top. Brush the pastry with water and sprinkle over the granulated sugar. Use a sharp knife to cut a few slashes in the top to allow steam to escape. Place the pie plate on a baking sheet and protect the crust edge with a ring made from foil.

❻ Bake for about 30 minutes until the crust is golden, then reduce the temperature to 180°C (350°F), Gas Mark 4 and bake for a further 30–40 minutes until the filling is bubbling and the pastry is crisp. Allow the pie to cool before serving.

MAPLE PECAN PIE

SERVES 6–8
PREPARATION TIME: 30 MINUTES,
PLUS COOLING AND CHILLING
COOKING TIME: 1 HOUR 15 MINUTES

300g (3 cups) pecans

75g (5 tablespoons) butter

100g (½ cup) light muscovado sugar

225g (generous ⅔ cup) golden syrup

225g (generous ⅔ cup) maple syrup

½ teaspoon salt

2 tablespoons bourbon whiskey (optional)

1 teaspoon apple cider vinegar

1 teaspoon vanilla extract

3 large eggs, beaten

Pastry

250g (2 cups) plain flour, plus extra
for dusting

125g (scant 1 cup) yellow cornmeal,
preferable stoneground

¼ teaspoon salt

250g (2¼ sticks) butter, cubed, plus extra
for greasing

150g (¾ cup) light muscovado sugar

finely grated zest of 1 lemon

3 large egg yolks

1 teaspoon vanilla extract

2 tablespoons water

❶ Preheat the oven to 180°C (350°F), Gas Mark 4. Spread the pecans on a baking sheet and toast for about 10 minutes until golden. Transfer to a plate to cool, then roughly crush half of them.

❷ For the pastry, place the flour, cornmeal and salt in a mixing bowl and stir to combine. Add the butter and rub in with the fingertips until the mixture resembles fine breadcrumbs. Stir in the sugar and lemon zest.

❸ Beat the egg yolks with the vanilla extract and measured water. Stir the liquid into the flour with a fork, then your fingers, and bring the mixture together to form a firm dough. Roll out the pastry on a lightly floured surface and use to line the base and sides of a greased 24-cm (9½-inch) pie dish. Trim the edges and chill in the refrigerator for at least 1 hour.

❹ Place the butter in a heavy-based saucepan over a medium heat with the sugar, golden syrup, maple syrup and salt. Bring to the boil, reduce the heat and simmer for 2 minutes, stirring. Remove from the heat and stir in the pecans, bourbon, if using, cider vinegar and vanilla extract. Pour the mixture into a bowl and set aside to cool for about 20 minutes, then beat in the eggs until well combined.

❺ Preheat the oven to 180°C (350°F), Gas Mark 4. Line the pastry case with baking paper and part-fill with baking beans. Bake blind for 15–20 minutes or until lightly golden, then remove the paper and beans. Reduce the temperature to 170°C (325°F), Gas Mark 3.

❻ Pour the filling mixture into the prepared pastry case and bake for a further 45–60 minutes or until the filling is just set. Serve warm.

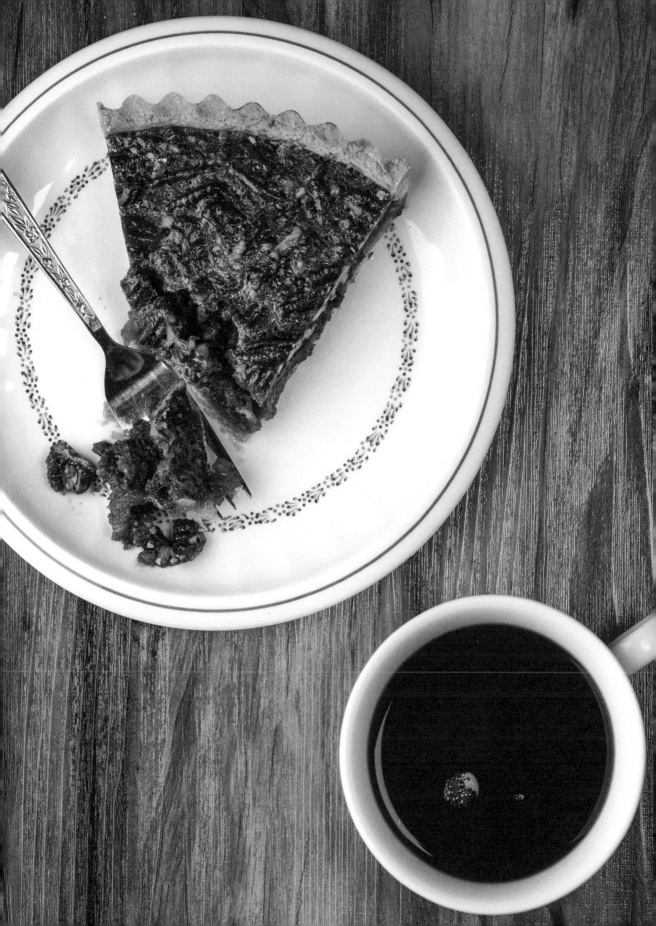

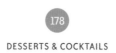
SWEET POTATO MERINGUE PIE

SERVES 6
PREPARATION TIME: 30 MINUTES,
PLUS CHILLING
COOKING TIME: 1 HOUR 5 MINUTES

1 quantity Sweet Shortcrust Pastry
(see page 181), chilled

flour, for dusting

butter, for greasing

500g (1lb 2oz) sweet potato, peeled
and diced

150ml (⅔ cup) double cream

75g (⅓ cup) light muscovado sugar

2 tablespoons runny honey

1 teaspoon ground ginger

1 teaspoon mixed spice

1 egg, plus 3 egg yolks

vanilla ice cream, to serve

Meringue topping

3 egg whites

50g (scant ¼ cup) light muscovado sugar

50g (¼ cup) caster sugar

½ teaspoon ground ginger

1 Preheat the oven to 180°C (350°F), Gas Mark 4. Roll out the pastry on a lightly floured surface and use to line the base and sides of a greased 20-cm (8-inch) pie dish. Trim the edges, then chill in the refrigerator for 15 minutes.

2 Place the sweet potato in the top of a steamer, cover and cook for 10 minutes or until tender. Mash with the cream, sugar, honey and spices, then beat in the whole egg and egg yolks. Pour into the pie case, level the surface, then bake for 40 minutes until set.

3 For the topping, place the egg whites in a clean, dry bowl and whisk until stiff peaks form. Gradually whisk in the sugars, a teaspoonful at a time, then add the ginger and whisk for a minute or two more until very thick and glossy. Spoon over the hot pie and swirl the meringue with the back of a spoon. Bake for 15 minutes until lightly browned and crisp.

4 Leave to cool for 30 minutes, then cut into wedges and serve warm with vanilla ice cream.

PUMPKIN PIE

SERVES 6
PREPARATION TIME: 30 MINUTES
COOKING TIME: 1–1¼ HOURS,
PLUS COOLING

500g (1lb 2oz) peeled and deseeded pumpkin or butternut squash, diced

3 eggs

100g (scant ½ cup) light muscovado sugar

2 tablespoons plain flour, plus extra for dusting

½ teaspoon ground cinnamon

½ teaspoon ground ginger

¼ teaspoon grated nutmeg

200ml (scant 1 cup) milk, plus extra to glaze

1 quantity Sweet Shortcrust Pastry (see page 181), chilled

butter, for greasing

icing sugar, for dusting

whipped cream, to serve

① Place the pumpkin in the top of a steamer, cover and cook for 15–20 minutes or until tender. Cool, then purée in a liquidizer or food processor.

② Place the eggs, sugar, flour and spices in a bowl and whisk until just mixed. Add the pumpkin purée, whisk until smooth, then gradually mix in the milk and set aside.

③ Preheat the oven to 190°C (375°F), Gas Mark 5. Roll out three-quarters of the pastry on a lightly floured surface and use to line a greased 23-cm (9-inch) enamel pie dish. Trim off the excess and add the trimmings to the reserved pastry. Roll out thinly and cut into tiny leaves, then mark with veins. Brush the pastry rim with milk, then press the leaves around the rim, reserving a few. Put the pie dish on a baking sheet.

④ Pour the pumpkin filling into the dish, decorate with a few more pastry leaves, then brush the pastry lightly with milk. Bake for 45–55 minutes until the filling is set and the pastry cooked through, covering with foil after 20 minutes if the pastry is becoming too brown.

⑤ Dust with a little icing sugar and serve with whipped cream.

CHOCOLATE CREAM PIE

SERVES 6–8
PREPARATION TIME: 30 MINUTES,
PLUS CHILLING AND COOLING
COOKING TIME: 45–50 MINUTES

1 quantity chocolate Shortcrust Pastry
(see opposite), made by replacing
2 tablespoons of the flour with
cocoa powder

butter, for greasing

150g (scant 1 cup) plain dark chocolate
(minimum 70% cocoa solids), chopped

500g (generous 2 cups) cream cheese,
softened

100g (½ cup) caster sugar

1 tablespoon plain flour, plus extra
for dusting

1 teaspoon vanilla extract

3 eggs

❶ Roll out the pastry on a lightly floured surface and use
to line a greased 23-cm (9-inch) fluted loose-bottomed
tart tin. Trim off the excess with scissors so it stands just
above the top of the tin. Prick the base with a fork, then chill
in the refrigerator for 15 minutes. Preheat the oven to 180°C
(350°F), Gas Mark 4.

❷ Line the pastry case with baking parchment and part-fill
with baking beans. Bake blind for 15 minutes, then remove
the paper and beans and cook for a further 5 minutes.
Reduce the oven temperature to 150°C (300°F), Gas Mark 2.

❸ Meanwhile, melt the chocolate in a heatproof bowl set
over a saucepan of gently simmering water, making sure the
water does not touch the bottom of the bowl. Place the cream
cheese in a separate bowl with the sugar, flour and vanilla
extract, then gradually beat in the eggs until smooth. Ladle
about one-third of the mixture into the chocolate bowl and
mix until smooth.

❹ Pour the vanilla cheese mixture into the tart case, then
pipe or spoon the chocolate mixture over the top and swirl
together with the handle of a teaspoon for a marbled effect.
Bake for a further 30–35 minutes until the edges of the filling
are set and beginning to crack, but the centre still wobbles
slightly. Leave to cool in the oven, then refrigerate overnight.
Serve in wedges.

PEACH MELBA PIE

SERVES 6
PREPARATION TIME: 40 MINUTES,
PLUS COOLING
COOKING TIME: 30–35 MINUTES

75g (1/3 cup) caster sugar, plus extra
for sprinkling

1 teaspoon cornflour

finely grated rind of 1 lemon

750g (1lb 10oz) peaches, skinned, pitted
and sliced

150g (1¼ cups) raspberries

milk, for glazing

Sweet shortcrust pastry

250g (2 cups) plain flour, plus extra
for dusting

50g (scant ¼ cup) caster sugar

pinch of salt

125g (1⅛ sticks) butter, diced, plus extra
for greasing

2½–3 tablespoons cold water

Melba sauce

200g (scant 1⅔ cups) raspberries

juice of ½ lemon

2 tablespoons icing sugar

❶ For the pastry, place the flour, sugar and salt in a mixing
bowl and stir to combine. Add the butter and rub in with
the fingertips until the mixture resembles fine breadcrumbs.
Gradually mix in just enough water to enable you to squeeze
the crumbs together to form a soft but not sticky dough.
Knead very lightly until smooth.

❷ Preheat the oven to 190°C (375°F), Gas Mark 5. Divide off
one-third of the pastry and set aside. Roll out the remaining
pastry on a lightly floured surface and use to line the base
and sides of a greased 20-cm (8-inch) pie dish.

❸ Mix the sugar, cornflour and lemon rind in a large bowl, then
add the fruits and toss together gently. Pile into the pie dish.

❹ Trim off the excess pastry, add to the reserved portion,
then roll it out. Cut into 1.5-cm (¾-inch) wide strips long
enough to go over the top of the pie. Brush the top edge of
the pie with milk and arrange the pastry strips over the top
as a lattice, pressing them on to the rim of the pie around
the edges. Trim off the excess pastry, brush with milk, then
sprinkle with a little sugar. Bake for 30–35 minutes until
golden, then allow to cool for 15 minutes.

❺ For the melba sauce, place all the ingredients in saucepan
over a medium heat and cook for 2–3 minutes until the
raspberries are just tender. Purée in a blender, then sieve to
remove the seeds. Serve the sauce warm or cold, drizzled
over wedges of the pie.

CONTRIBUTED BY
CAST MEMBER
**KIMMY
ROBERTSON**

182

DESSERTS & COCKTAILS

ANGEL FOOD CAKE

Deputy Andy Brennan's favourite dessert, as imagined by cast-member Kimmy Robertson, who played his girlfriend "Lucy Moran".

One of our favourite couples from *Twin Peaks* has to be loyal Sheriff's receptionist Lucy Moran and her on/off boyfriend – and the potential father of her baby – Deputy Andy Brennan.

Lucy is portrayed by the charming actress Kimmy Robertson. Here she imagines an episode in Lucy and Andy's life.

First...go to the grocery store and buy a Van de Kamp's Bakery Angel Food Cake. Be sure to get the round one with the hole in the middle...not the rectangular one that doesn't even look like a cake but more like a doorstop. And who wants to eat a doorstop? Nobody.

Second...while you are there. pick up a can of Duncan Hines Milk Chocolate Home-style Frosting.

When you get home be sure to take the cake out of the package and transfer it to your prettiest cake stand with the matching lid. Whichever one you have left that the housekeeper hasn't smashed into bits.

Open the can of icing and be sure to put the plastic lid into the correct recycling bin. You will be using every molecule of this delicious icing. Then get a nice smooth table-knife and stir up the chocolate icing until it is creamy and looks like homemade. Spread the icing all over the cake and don't forget the hole. When it is all covered. use the knife to make little curlicues all over the beautiful cake.

Cover and place in a part of the kitchen where your Love will be sure to see it when they walk in...you will get a kiss for this.

As far as the milk is concerned...Andy buys ours from a local farmer named Mr Champ (not his real name). They have to meet in the alley. Oh well. I can't reveal which alley because. as you know. raw. fresh-squeezed organic milk is illegal in every state but California. But we won't speak about the indiscretions of the United States Government as Andy has a pension coming.

Now go and put on your best lounge wear—Andy loves me in a pink satin bathrobe with matching slippers—and have a beautiful evening.

Love.
Lucy xx

NADINE HURLEY'S MARSHMALLOW COTTON BALLS

MAKES ABOUT 60
PREPARATION TIME: 50 MINUTES
COOKING TIME: 50 MINUTES

6 tablespoons icing sugar

6 tablespoons cornflour

450g (2¼ cups) caster sugar

1 tablespoon liquid glucose

200ml (scant 1 cup) water

8 sheets of gelatine, about 13g (½oz) in total

2 large egg whites

pinch of salt

1 teaspoon vanilla extract

50g (½ cup) hazelnuts or pecans

150g (scant 1 cup) plain dark chocolate (minimum 70% cocoa solids), chopped

❶ Sieve the icing sugar and cornflour into a bowl. Line 2 baking sheets with baking parchment and dust liberally with the icing sugar and cornflour mixture.

❷ Place the caster sugar, glucose and water into a heavy-based saucepan over a medium heat and bring to the boil, stirring to dissolve the sugar. Reduce the heat and simmer gently, without stirring, for 20–30 minutes until the mixture reaches 115–120°C (235–250°F) on a sugar thermometer. If you don't have a sugar thermometer, drop a little of the syrup into a cup of water to cool. It should form a soft ball which can be moulded with the fingers.

❸ Meanwhile, soak the gelatine in a large bowl of cold water for about 10 minutes until wobbly and soft.

❹ Place the egg whites and salt in a really clean bowl and whisk with a free-standing mixer or hand-held electric mixer until stiff and glossy. Gradually add the hot syrup, whisking all the time until thoroughly incorporated.

❺ Lift the gelatine out of the bowl and squeeze gently in your hands to remove any excess water. Place it in the hot syrup pan and roll around until melted, then gradually beat this into the meringue mixture. Add the vanilla extract and continue whisking for 5–10 minutes until the marshmallow has almost completely cooled.

6 Place spoonfuls of the marshmallow mixture on the lined sheets and dust liberally with more of the icing sugar and cornflour mixture. Leave overnight to set.

7 Preheat the oven to 180°C (350°F), Gas Mark 4. Spread the nuts out on a baking sheet and toast for 5–10 minutes or until golden. Transfer to a plate to cool, then chop them finely.

8 Melt the chocolate in a heatproof bowl set over a saucepan of gently simmering water, making sure the water does not touch the bottom of the bowl. Skewer some of the marshmallows on wooden candy sticks (or curtain track!), dip into the chocolate, then sprinkle some with chopped nuts. Keep some of the marshmallows plain. Arrange on a baking sheet lined with baking parchment and leave until set.

See photograph overleaf.

As well as playing husband and wife in *Twin Peaks*, Everett McGill and Wendy Robie (Ed and Nadine Hurley) teamed up again in the 1992 Wes Craven horror film, *The People Under the Stairs*.

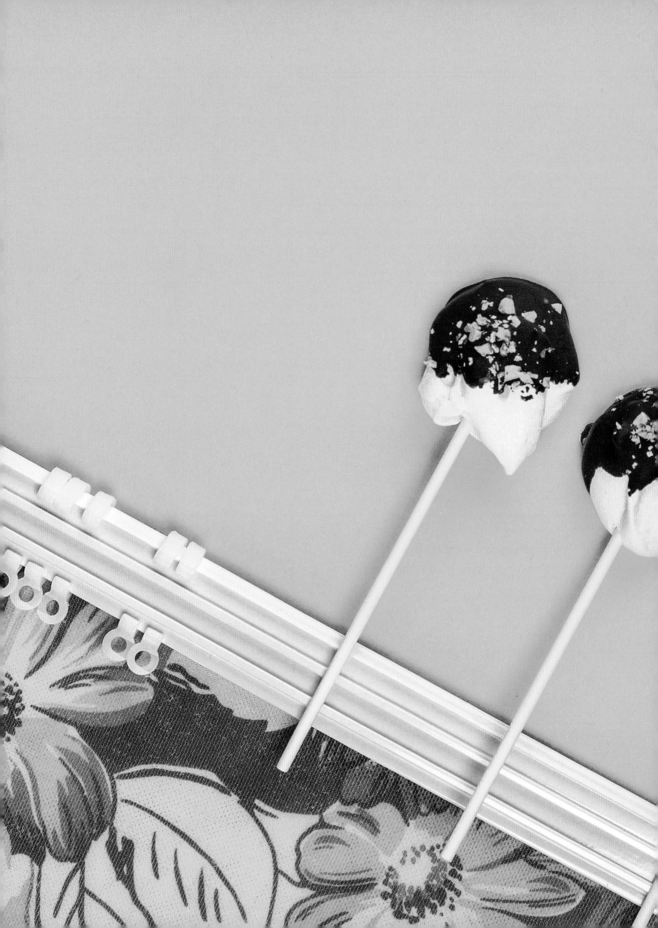

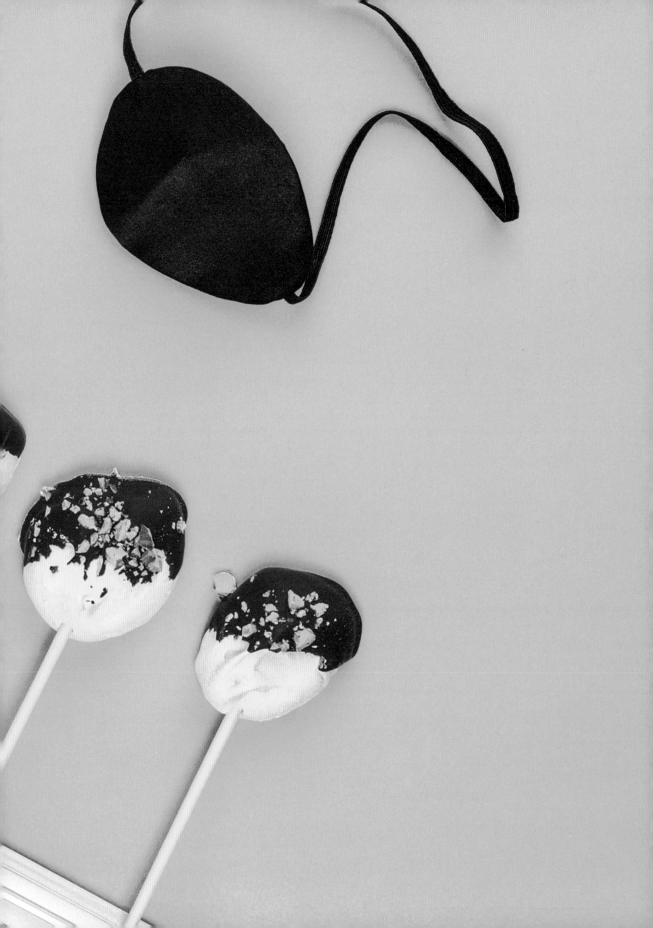

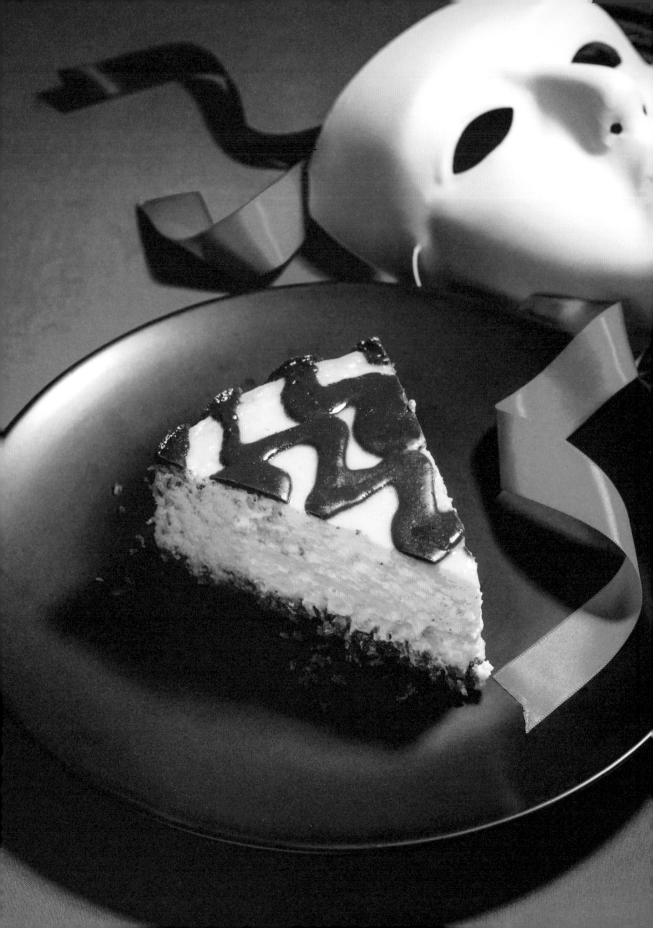

COCONUT CHEESECAKE

SERVES 8–10
PREPARATION TIME: 40 MINUTES
COOKING TIME: 1½–2 HOURS

900g (4 cups) full-fat cream cheese,
at room temperature

250g (1¼ cups) caster sugar

4 large eggs

400-ml (14-oz) can coconut milk

1 teaspoon vanilla extract

juice of 1 lemon

150g (1⅔ cups) desiccated coconut

2½ tablespoons cornflour

pinch of salt

Chocolate chevrons

100ml (scant ½ cup) double cream

75g (scant ½ cup) plain dark chocolate
(minimum 70% cocoa solids), chopped

Base

100g (3½oz) digestive biscuits

150g (1⅜ sticks) unsalted butter, melted

2 tablespoons cocoa powder

100g (generous 1 cup) desiccated coconut

pinch of salt

❶ For the chocolate chevrons, place the cream in a small saucepan over a medium heat and bring to the boil. Remove from the heat, add the chocolate and stir until melted. Transfer to a bowl and place in the refrigerator to cool and thicken, beating it from time to time. It needs to be thick enough to drizzle and hold a line, but not set hard.

❷ Preheat the oven to 180°C (350°F), Gas Mark 4. Place the biscuits in a plastic bag and bash with a rolling pin into fine crumbs. Transfer to a bowl and add the melted butter, cocoa powder, coconut and salt.

❸ Press the mixture evenly into the bottom of a 23–24-cm (9–9½-inch) spring-form cake tin. Bake for 10 minutes, then leave to cool. Increase the heat to 240°C (475°F), Gas Mark 9.

❹ Place the cream cheese in a bowl with the sugar and beat until smooth. Add the eggs, coconut milk, vanilla extract and lemon juice and beat until well blended. Stir in the desiccated coconut, cornflour and salt.

❺ Pour the mixture into the cake tin on top of the biscuit base and bake for 10 minutes. Carefully remove from the oven and reduce the heat to 120°C (250°F), Gas Mark ½.

❻ Using a flat piping nozzle, pipe or drizzle the chocolate mixture over the cheesecake to make the chevron pattern. Return to the oven and bake for a further 1–1½ hours until just set but still a little wobbly in the middle. Turn off the oven but leave the cheesecake inside to cool. When completely cold, cover and refrigerate overnight.

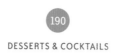
DONNA HAYWARD'S COFFEE & WHITE CHOCOLATE CRÈME BRÛLÉE

SERVES 6
PREPARATION TIME: 15 MINUTES
COOKING TIME: 50 MINUTES

25g (⅓ cup) coffee beans

500ml (generous 2 cups) double cream

50g (scant ¼ cup) soft light brown sugar,
plus extra for sprinkling

75g (scant ½ cup) white chocolate,
finely chopped

2 egg yolks

❶ Preheat the oven to 180°C (350°F), Gas Mark 4. Spread the coffee beans on a baking sheet and toast for 10 minutes. Allow to cool.

❷ Place the cream and sugar in a heavy-based saucepan over a medium heat and bring to the boil, stirring to dissolve the sugar. Remove from the heat and stir in the chocolate until melted, then add the coffee beans. Cover and leave to infuse for 30 minutes.

❸ Preheat the oven to 150°C (300°F), Gas Mark 2. Whisk the egg yolks in a bowl until pale in colour, then pour the cream mixture through a sieve into the bowl, whisking continuously until smooth.

❹ Divide the mixture between 6 heatproof ramekins, about 100ml (scant ½ cup) each. Stand the ramekins in a roasting tin and pour enough boiling water into the tin to come halfway up their sides. Bake for about 30 minutes until almost set, but still a little wobbly in the middle. Leave to cool, then chill in the refrigerator until very cold.

❺ Sprinkle the tops of the ramekins with an even layer of brown sugar, then use a blow torch to melt and caramelize this. Alternatively, preheat a grill to very high and place the ramekins under it to caramelize the sugar. Let the caramel harden, then return the crème brûlées to the refrigerator until you are ready to serve them.

MARGARET LANTERMAN'S CHOCOLATE CHESTNUT LOG

SERVES 8
PREPARATION TIME: 35 MINUTES
COOKING TIME: 15 MINUTES

50g (generous ¼ cup) plain dark chocolate (minimum 70% cocoa solids), chopped

4 egg whites

pinch of salt

200g (1 cup) golden caster sugar, plus extra for sprinkling

cocoa powder, for dusting

Filling

200g (generous 1⅓ cups) canned or vac-packed chestnuts, roughly chopped

2 heaped tablespoons icing sugar

1 teaspoon vanilla extract

pinch of salt

250g (generous 1 cup) mascarpone

200ml (scant 1 cup) double cream

50g (generous ¼ cup) plain dark chocolate (minimum 70% cocoa solids), roughly chopped

❶ Preheat the oven to 180°C (350°F), Gas Mark 4 and line a 23 x 30-cm (9 x 12-inch) Swiss roll tin with baking parchment. Melt the chocolate in a heatproof bowl set over a saucepan of gently simmering water, making sure the water does not touch the bottom of the bowl.

❷ Place the egg whites and salt in a large mixing bowl and whisk until soft peaks form. Whisk in the caster sugar, a spoonful at a time, until the mixture is stiff and glossy.

❸ Drizzle a little of the melted chocolate backwards and forwards over the meringue in the bowl, then spoon the meringue evenly over the lined Swiss roll tin, drizzling more chocolate into the bowl each time you take out a spoonful of meringue.

❹ Carefully spread the meringue out evenly and drizzle any remaining chocolate over the surface. Bake for 15 minutes until crisp on the outside. Allow to cool completely.

❺ Lay a sheet of baking parchment on the work surface and sprinkle evenly with caster sugar. Turn the cooled meringue out on to the paper and carefully peel the lining paper away from the meringue.

❻ For the filling, place the chestnuts in the bowl of a food processor with the icing sugar, vanilla extract and salt and blend until smooth. Transfer the mixture to a large bowl and stir in the mascarpone.

❼ Whip the cream until soft peaks form, then fold it into the chestnut mixture with half of the chopped chocolate. Spread the filling over the meringue and roll up the log, using the paper to support it while you roll. Dust lightly with cocoa powder, sprinkle with the remaining chopped chocolate, and serve in slices.

See photograph overleaf

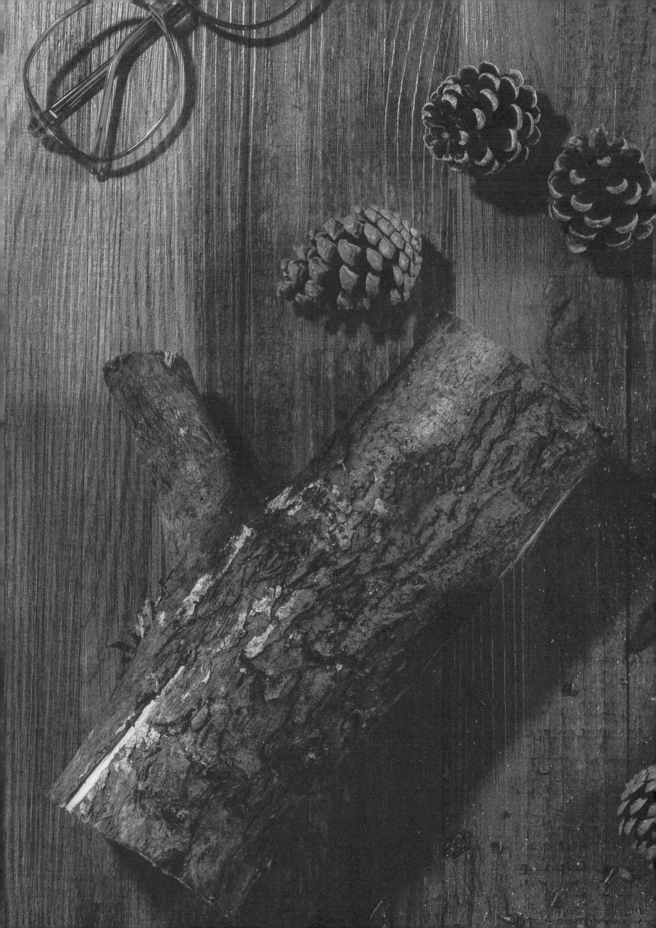

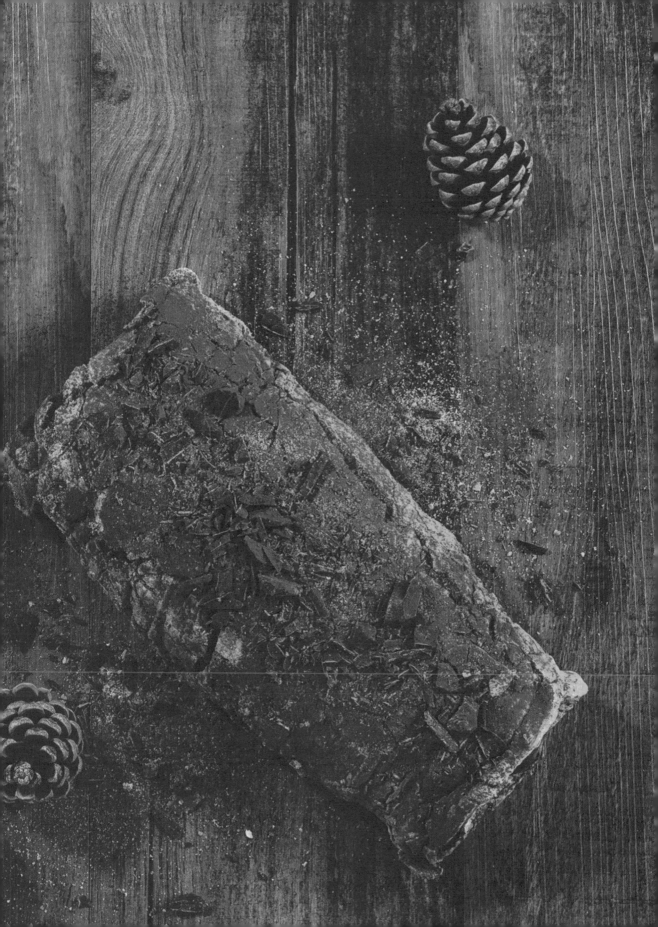

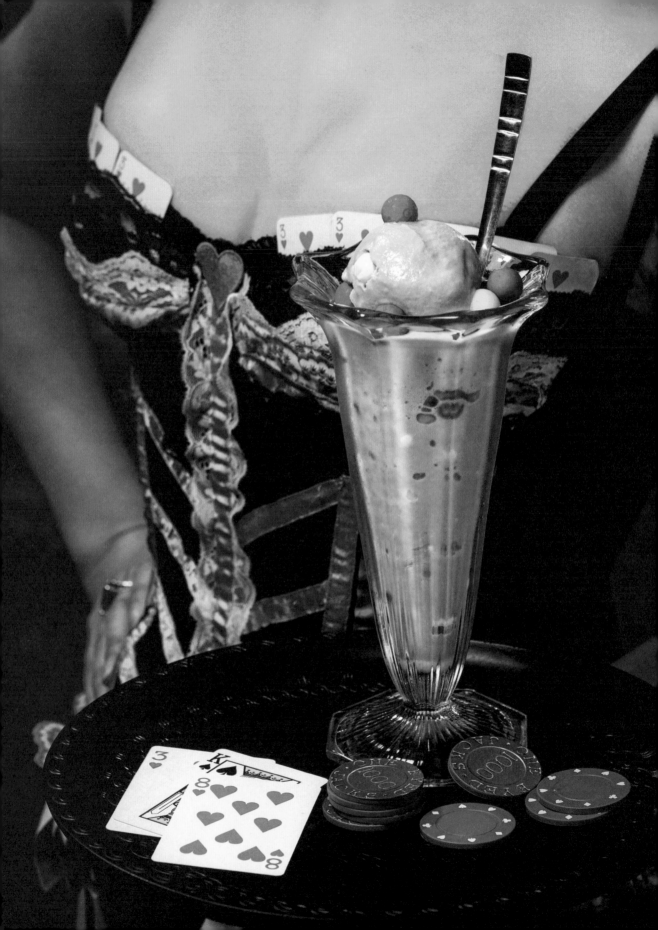

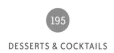
LELAND PALMER'S BUBBLEGUM ICE CREAM

SERVES 6–8
PREPARATION TIME: 10 MINUTES,
PLUS CHILLING AND FREEZING
COOKING TIME: 25 MINUTES

600ml (2½ cups) double cream

75g (2¾oz) bubblegum

1 teaspoon vanilla extract

5 large egg yolks

200g (1 cup) caster sugar

pinch of salt

blue food colouring

150g (5½oz) small mixed gum balls

❶ Place the cream in a heavy-based saucepan over a medium heat until almost boiling. Remove from the heat, stir in the bubblegum and vanilla extract and leave to infuse for 1 hour.

❷ Place the egg yolks, sugar and salt in a large bowl and beat until smooth. Pour the cream into the bowl through a sieve and whisk until combined. Return the mixture to the saucepan and place over a very low heat. Stir constantly until the custard has thickened, taking care not to let it get too hot or it will curdle.

❸ Pour through a sieve into a clean bowl, stir in several drops of food colouring, then place cling film on the surface to stop a skin forming. Allow to cool, then chill completely in the refrigerator.

❹ Churn the custard in an ice-cream machine until frozen, or pour into a plastic container and place in the freezer until frozen, beating the mixture every 30 minutes until smooth. Stir in the gum balls and store in the freezer until ready to serve.

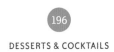

LIL'S BLUE ROSE CUPCAKES

MAKES 16
PREPARATION TIME: 45 MINUTES
COOKING TIME: 15–20 MINUTES

180g (1½ cups) self-raising flour

1 teaspoon baking powder

pinch of salt

180g (1⅝ sticks) unsalted butter, softened

180g (generous ¾ cup) caster sugar

1 teaspoon rosewater

3 large eggs

Frosting

200g (scant 1 cup) cream cheese

100g (7 tablespoons) unsalted butter, softened

600g (5 cups) icing sugar

1 teaspoon rosewater

blue food colouring

❶ Preheat the oven to 180°C (350°F), Gas Mark 4 and line 2 12-hole cupcake trays with 16 paper cases. Sift the flour, baking powder and salt into a bowl.

❷ Place the butter, sugar and rosewater in a separate large bowl and beat until very smooth. Add the eggs, one at a time, beating well after each addition and adding some flour halfway through if necessary to prevent curdling, then gently fold in the flour mixture until well combined.

❸ Divide the mixture evenly between the paper cases and bake for 15–20 minutes until risen and golden. Remove from the oven and leave to cool in the tin for 5 minutes, then transfer to a wire rack to cool completely.

❹ For the frosting, place the cream cheese, butter, icing sugar and rosewater in a mixing bowl and beat until light and fluffy. Add a few drops of blue food colouring until you reach the desired shade.

❺ Once the cupcakes are completely cold, spoon the icing into a piping bag fitted with a 2d flower nozzle and use to ice the cakes to look like roses.

SALTINES WITH APPLE BUTTER

MAKES ABOUT 50
PREPARATION TIME: 30 MINUTES
COOKING TIME: 3–4 HOURS

300g (scant 2½ cups) plain flour, plus extra for dusting

2 teaspoons baking powder

pinch of salt

50g (3½ tablespoons) unsalted butter, cubed

125ml (½ cup) milk

1 egg yolk

1 tablespoon water

sea salt flakes, for sprinkling

smoked cheese, to serve

Apple butter

1.5kg (3lb 5oz) apples, peeled, cored and quartered

200ml (scant 1 cup) unfiltered apple juice

150g (generous ⅔ cup cup) light muscovado sugar

finely grated zest and juice of 2 lemons

1 vanilla pod, split lengthways

½ teaspoon salt

1 teaspoon ground cinnamon

1 teaspoon ground ginger

½ teaspoon ground cardamom

½ nutmeg, finely grated

¼ teaspoon ground mace

❶ Place the apples a large saucepan over a high heat and add the apple juice, sugar, lemon zest and juice, vanilla pod and salt. Bring to the boil, reduce the heat and simmer, half covered, for about 20 minutes or until the apples are soft and tender.

❷ Remove the apples from the heat and stir in all of the spices. Leave to cool for 10 minutes, then use a stick blender to blend until smooth.

❸ Preheat the oven to 150°C (300°F), Gas Mark 2. Transfer the apple mixture to an ovenproof dish and bake, uncovered, for 2½–3½ hours, stirring every 30 minutes, until thick and deep amber in colour. Allow to cool completely, then store in an airtight container until ready to use.

❹ Preheat the oven to 200°C (400°F), Gas Mark 6 and line 2 baking sheets with baking parchment.

❺ Place the flour and salt in a mixing bowl and stir to combine. Add the butter and rub in with the fingertips until the mixture resembles fine breadcrumbs, then stir through the baking powder.

❻ Slowly add the milk until the mixture forms a soft but firm dough. Divide the dough in half and roll out each piece on a lightly floured work surface to 2–3mm (1/12–1/10 inch) thick. Cut the dough into 5-cm (2-inch) squares using a large sharp knife or pastry roller. Reroll any trimmings and cut again.

❼ Transfer the squares to the lined sheets and pierce each cracker evenly with a fork to create small holes. Beat the egg yolk with the measured water and brush evenly over the crackers. Sprinkle with a few sea salt flakes, then bake for 6–8 minutes until lightly golden. Allow to cool, then serve with smoked cheese and the apple butter.

LAURA PALMER'S SILK STOCKING

MAKES 1

———

drinking chocolate powder

¾ measure tequila

¾ measure white crème de cacao

3½ measures single cream

2 teaspoons grenadine

ice cubes

❶ Dampen the rim of a chilled martini glass and dip it into a saucer of drinking chocolate powder.

❷ Pour the tequila, crème de cacao, cream and grenadine into a cocktail shaker with some ice cubes and shake until a frost forms on the outside of the shaker. Strain into the prepared glass and serve.

JOSIE PACKARD'S FIFTH AVENUE

MAKES 1

———

1 measure crème de cacao

1 measure apricot brandy

1 measure single cream

❶ Pour the crème de cacao into a straight-sided shot glass. Using the back of a bar spoon, slowly float the apricot brandy over the crème de cacao to form a separate layer.

❷ Layer the cream over the apricot brandy in the same way and serve.

HANK JENNINGS' BEETNICK

MAKES 1

1½ measures vodka

1 measure beetroot juice

1 measure orange juice

2 teaspoons lemon juice

1 teaspoon agave syrup

ice cubes

orange twist, to decorate

1 Pour the vodka, beetroot, orange and lemon juices and agave syrup into a cocktail shaker with some ice cubes and shake until a frost forms on the outside of the shaker.

2 Strain into a martini glass, decorate with an orange twist and serve.

CATHERINE MARTELL'S SAPPHIRE MARTINI

MAKES 1

2 measures gin

½ measure blue Curaçao

ice cubes

red or blue cocktail cherry, to decorate

1 Pour the gin and blue Curaçao into a cocktail shaker with some ice cubes and shake until a frost forms on the outside of the shaker.

2 Strain into a martini glass, carefully drop a cherry into the glass and serve.

ESPRESSO MARTINI

MAKES 1

1 measure coffee liqueur

1 measure espresso

4 measures of vodka

ice cubes

3 coffee beans, to decorate

❶ Pour the coffee liqueur, espresso and vodka into a cocktail shaker with some ice cubes and shake until a frost forms on the outside of the shaker.

❷ Strain into a chilled cocktail glass and decorate with the coffee beans.

EGG NOG

MAKES 1

1 measure brandy

1 measure dark rum

1 egg

1 teaspoon sugar syrup

ice cubes

3 measures full-fat milk

freshly grated nutmeg, to decorate

❶ Pour the brandy, rum, egg and sugar syrup into a cocktail shaker with some ice cubes and shake until a frost forms on the outside of the shaker.

❷ Strain into a toddy glass and pour over the milk. Decorate with a little grated nutmeg and serve.

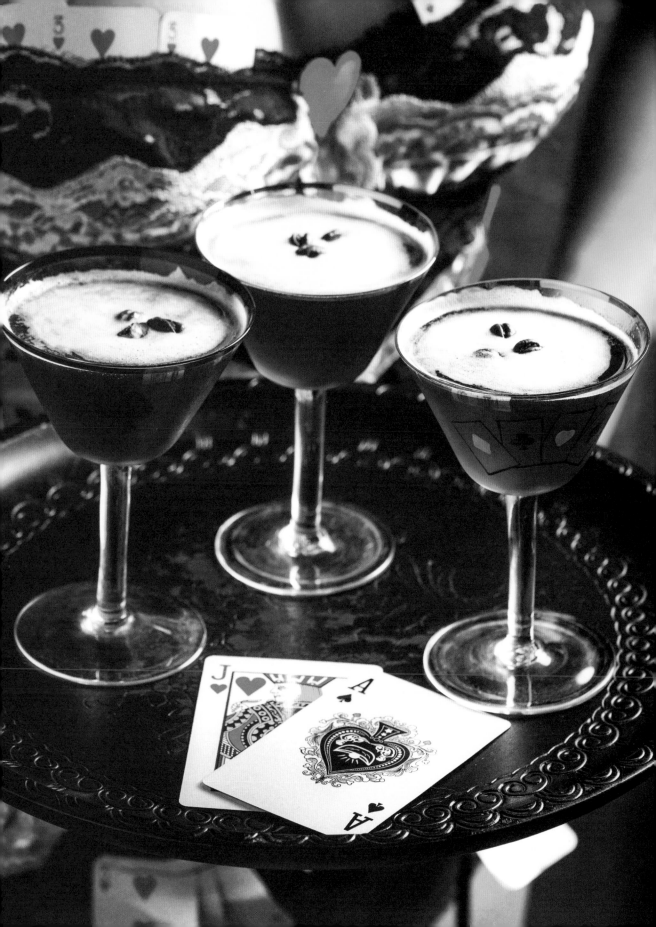

TIKI TREAT

MAKES 1

crushed ice

½ ripe mango, peeled and pitted, plus extra slices to decorate

3 chunks of fresh coconut

1 measure coconut cream

2 measures aged rum

1 dash of lemon juice

1 teaspoon caster sugar

1 Put a small scoop of crushed ice with all the other ingredients into a food processor or blender and blend until smooth.

2 Pour into a hurricane glass, decorate with mango slices and serve with a straw.

FLAMING LAMBORGHINI

MAKES 1

1 measure Kahlúa coffee liqueur

1 measure Sambuca

1 measure Bailey's Irish Cream

1 measure blue Curaçao

1 Pour the Kahlúa into a warmed martini glass. Using the back of a bar spoon, slowly float half the Sambuca over the Kahlúa to form a separate layer.

2 Pour the Bailey's and Curaçao into shot glasses.

3 Next, pour the remaining Sambuca into a warmed wine glass and set it alight. Carefully pour it into the martini glass.

4 Pour the Bailey's and Curaçao into the lit martini glass at the same time. Serve with straws.

TOM COLLINS

MAKES 1

———

2 measures gin

1 measure sugar syrup

1 measure lemon juice

ice cubes

4 measures soda water

To decorate

lemon wedge

black cherry

❶ Pour the gin, sugar syrup and lemon juice into a cocktail shaker with some ice cubes and shake until a frost forms on the outside of the shaker.

❷ Strain into a Collins glass full of ice cubes and top up with the soda water. Decorate with a lemon wedge and a cherry and serve.

GODMOTHER

MAKES 1

———

cracked ice cubes

1½ measures vodka

½ measure Amaretto di Saronno

❶ Put 2–3 cracked ice cubes in an old-fashioned glass. Add the vodka and Amaretto, stir lightly to mix and serve.

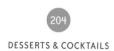
JUDGE STERNWOOD'S YUCKON SUCKER PUNCH WITH AUDREY'S KISS

MAKES 1

1½ measures bourbon whiskey

½ measure coffee liqueur

3 measures strong espresso coffee

ice cubes

soda water, to top up

2 tablespoons double cream

dash of blue Curaçao

1 maraschino cherry with a stalk

❶ Pour the bourbon, coffee liqueur and espresso into a mixing glass with some ice cubes and stir well. Strain into a tall, narrow glass and top up with soda water until the glass is three-quarters full.

❷ Meanwhile, lightly whip the cream with the Curaçao until thickened. Using the back of a bar spoon, slowly float the cream on top of the drink to make a separate layer. Decorate with a kiss from Miss Audrey Horne (a cherry with a stalk).

BENJAMIN HORNE'S OLD-FASHIONED

MAKES 1

ice cubes

2 measures bourbon whiskey

1 teaspoon sugar syrup

1 dash of orange bitters

1 dash of Angostura bitters

orange twist, to decorate

❶ Half-fill an old-fashioned glass with ice cubes. Add the remaining ingredients to the glass and stir for 1 minute.

❷ Fill the glass with more ice cubes, decorate with an orange twist and serve.

RONETTE PULASKI'S SWEET & CHILLI

MAKES 1

1½ measures Scotch whisky

¾ measure blood orange juice

¾ measure Antica Formula or sweet vermouth

1 teaspoon agave syrup

ice cubes

1 red chilli, about 2.5cm (1 inch) long, to decorate

❶ Pour the whisky, blood orange juice, Antica Formula or vermouth and agave syrup into a cocktail shaker with some ice cubes and shake until a frost forms on the outside of the shaker.

❷ Strain into a frozen coupette or margarita glass, decorate with a chilli and serve.

DICK TREMAYNE'S SCOTCH GINGER HIGHBALL

MAKES 1

---

ice cubes

2 measures Scotch whisky

1 measure lemon juice

3 teaspoons sugar syrup

4 measures ginger ale

1 slice of fresh root ginger, to decorate

❶ Fill a highball glass with ice cubes. Pour over the whisky, lemon juice, sugar syrup and ginger ale and stir. Decorate with a slice of fresh root ginger and serve.

AUDREY HORNE'S AMERICAN BELLE

MAKES 1

½ measure cherry liqueur
½ measure Amaretto di Saronno
½ measure bourbon whiskey

❶ Pour the cherry liqueur into a shot glass. Using the back of a bar spoon, slowly float the Amaretto over the cherry liqueur to form a separate layer.

❷ Layer the bourbon over the Amaretto in the same way and serve.

AUDREY HORNE'S CHERRY JULEP

MAKES 1

juice of ½ lemon
1 teaspoon sugar syrup
1 teaspoon grenadine
1 measure cherry brandy
1 measure sloe gin
2 measures gin
ice cubes, plus crushed ice to serve
lemon rind strips, to decorate

❶ Pour the lemon juice, sugar syrup, grenadine, cherry brandy, sloe gin and gin into a cocktail shaker with some ice cubes and shake until a frost forms on the outside of the shaker.

❷ Fill a highball glass with crushed ice, strain the drink over the top, decorate with lemon rind strips and serve.

HOW TO TIE A CHERRY STEM LIKE AUDREY HORNE

One of every Peakie's favourite scenes is where Audrey Horne seductively ties a cherry stem in her mouth using only her tongue, to gain a job at One Eyed Jacks. Let's be honest, we've all tried it and failed. But fear not! Now you can become master of the cherry stem by following the simple instructions below. You'll be the envy of your friends at every Peakie party!

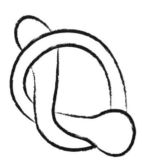

You will need

1 fresh Morello cherry with stem, ends intact

1 strong tongue

Method

1 Eat the cherry, all the time confidently holding the eye of your suitor.

2 Pop the cherry stem in your mouth in a slow seductive manner and use your tongue to bend it one-third of the way along its length so you have two sides, one longer than the other. Make sure the shorter end crosses the longer end.

3 Use your tongue to turn the stem around so that the longer part of the stem is on the bottom and the ends point towards the back of your mouth.

4 Using your tongue and the back of your teeth, push the loop upwards and flip it as though towards the back of your mouth while pressing it towards your front top teeth.

5 Use your tongue to push the end of the longer part of the stem through the loop and secure it in the middle of the loop (this is the part where you'll probably stop looking seductive!).

6 Take the perfectly tied cherry stem from your mouth in a provocative manner. See, easy isn't it?

BEDTIME BOUNCER

MAKES 1

2 measures brandy
1 measure Cointreau
5 measures bitter lemon
ice cubes
lemon spiral, to decorate

❶ Pour the brandy, Cointreau and bitter lemon into a mixing glass and stir well.

❷ Place 4–6 ice cubes in a highball glass and pour the brandy mixture over the ice. Decorate with a lemon spiral and serve with a straw.

GRASSHOPPER

MAKES 1

1 measure white crème de cacao
1 measure crème de menthe
mint sprig, to decorate

❶ Pour the crème de cacao into a martini glass.

❷ Using the back of a bar spoon, slowly float the crème de menthe over the crème de cacao to form a separate layer. Decorate with a mint sprig and serve.

FIREBALL

MAKES 1

½ measure absinthe

½ measure ice-cold kümmel

½ measure Goldschläger

1 Pour the absinthe into a shot glass. Using the back of a bar spoon, slowly float the kümmel over the absinthe to form a separate layer.

2 Layer the Goldschläger over the kümmel in the same way and serve.

GLÖGG

SERVES 8–10

1 bottle dry red wine, or ½ bottle red wine and ½ bottle port or Madeira

pared rind of ½ orange

10 cardamom pods, lightly crushed

1 cinnamon stick

10 whole cloves

75g (generous ½ cup) blanched almonds

125g (scant 1 cup) raisins

125–175g (4–6oz) sugar cubes

150ml (⅔ cup) Aquavit or brandy

1 Pour the wine, or wine and port or Madeira, into a saucepan. Tie the orange rind and spices in a piece of muslin and add to the pan. Add the almonds and raisins. Heat at just below boiling point for 25 minutes, stirring occasionally.

2 Place a wire rack over the saucepan and arrange the sugar cubes on it. Warm the Aquavit or brandy and pour it over the sugar cubes to saturate them evenly. Set them alight: they will melt through the wire rack into the wine.

3 Stir the glögg and remove the spice bag. Serve hot, with a few raisins and almonds in each cup.

ABOUT THE AUTHOR
TWIN PEAKS *UK FESTIVAL*

The author of this cookbook, Lindsey Bowden, founded the *Twin Peaks* UK Festival in 2010. Originally intended as a one-off for the 20th Anniversary of *Twin Peaks*, the festival has grown into something very special and continues to be a sell-out success to this day. In 2015 the festival was extended to a weekend event to celebrate the 25th Anniversary of the show and included a full-size train car and a re-enactment of the murder of Laura Palmer.

The festival is a celebration of *Twin Peaks* and all things Lynch and immerses fans in that strange and wonderful world. It includes screenings, performances, guests from the show and much more. The festival is heavily focused on how the fans are inspired by *Twin Peaks* and features a popular art gallery and a Lynch Inspired Short Films section. It also recreates sets from the show, allowing fans to dive fully into the world of *Twin Peaks*.

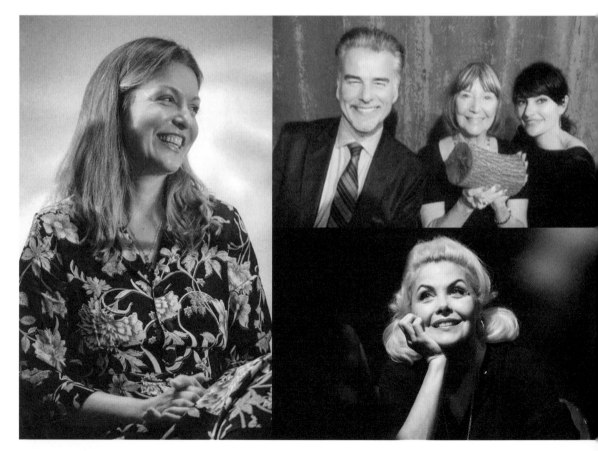

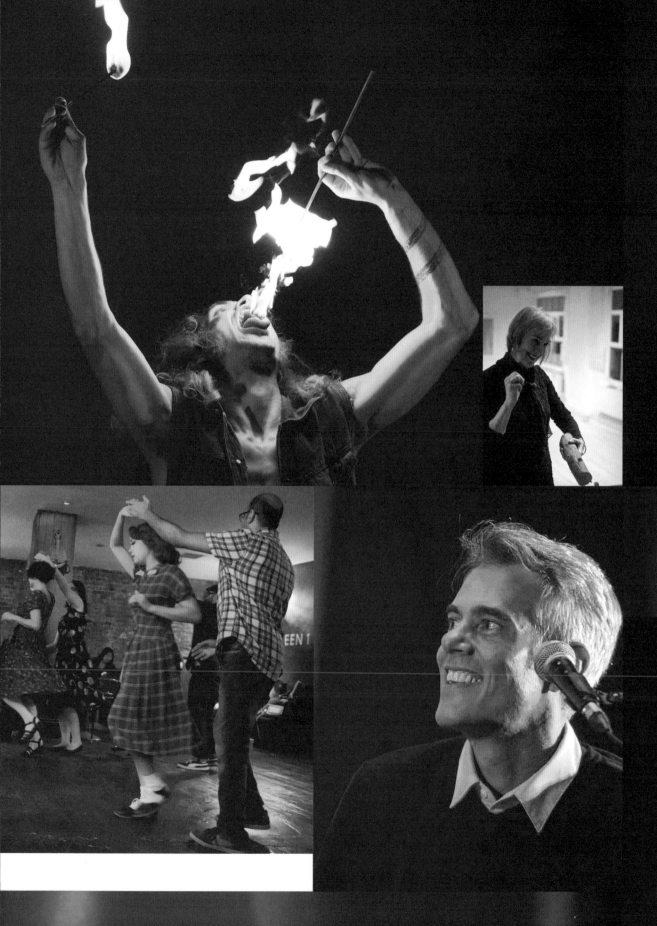

THE DOUBLE R CLUB

"This evening of mystery and nightmares inspired by the films of David Lynch is a dark and twisted treat, often groping into territory where other cabaret nights fear to tread."

TimeOut

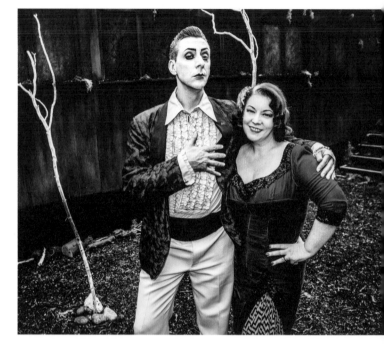

The Double R Club has been closely associated with the annual *Twin Peaks* UK Festival since its inception in 2010 and has contributed recipes to this cookbook. Founded in 2009, Club is the brainchild of Rose Thorne and Benjamin Louche. The aim is to present cabaret in a less frivolous way, a way that may even disturb and disquiet, or perhaps conjure up bad dreams. The worlds of David Lynch seemed like the perfect catalyst.

The Double R has twice won 'Best Ongoing Production' at the London Cabaret Awards, as well as The Erotic Award for 'Best Club/Event'. Additionally Benjamin Louche won 'Best Host' at the 2014 London Cabaret Awards.

"The Double R Club is a terrifying yet addictive experience that will send you on a portentous rollercoaster and leave you begging for sweet mercy by the end! If you are looking for a frivolous joyful evening then the Double R Club is not for you."

21st Century Burlesque

With huge thanks to The Double R Club performers who have performed at the **Twin Peaks** *UK Festival since our beginning in 2010.*

Benjamin Louche

Rose Thorne

Heavy Metal Pete

Miss Miranda

Lydia Darling

Snake Fervor

Laurence Owen

Randolph Hott

Em Brulee

Hotcake Kitty

Tallulah Mockingbird

VJ Spankie

Kiki Lovechild

Emerald Fontaine

Des O' Connor

Nara Queen of the Night

The Dr. Jacoby Experience

Greasy Tony

Torch Song Tilly G

Miss Giddy Heights & The
    Doppelgangers

Twice Shy Theatre

Eliza DeLite

Nathan Dean Williams

And thanks to the wonderful 52 Card Pick Up Girls

Louise Holland

Yvonne Holland

Abbi De Carteret-Feazey

Mina Dutton

Ruth Young

And the **Twin Peaks** *UK Festival manicurists*

Jo Walsh

Hellen Burrough

Lain Freefall

And the wonderful Sean 'Magic' Mooney

Catch The Double R Club every month at Bethnal Green Working Men's Club.

www.thedoublerclub.co.uk

"London can't claim too many shows with the impressive longevity and sheer depravity of the East-End based Double R Club." **Londonist**

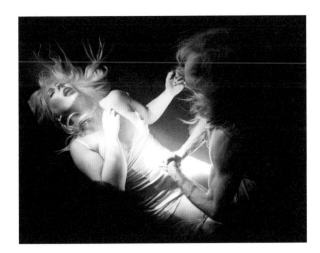

THE BIG DONUT QUIZ ANSWERS

ANSWER 1   10 billion.

ANSWER 2   Jelly donuts.

ANSWER 3   "Harry, that goes without saying."

ANSWER 4   10.

ANSWER 5   20.

ANSWER 6   In the Sheriff's station wagon.

ANSWER 7   In the kitchenette in the lobby of the Sheriff's station in pink boxes.

ANSWER 8   Father Christmas.

ANSWER 9   Deputy "Hawk", Gordon Cole, Agent Dale Cooper, Deputy Andy Brennan and Sheriff Truman.

ANSWER 10   12.

ANSWER 11   "Forgive my saying so Catherine, but aren't you dead?"

ANSWER 12   A large pile of logs.

ANSWER 13   1920.

ANSWER 14   "A policeman's dream".

ANSWER 15   Boston.

GLOSSARY OF COOKING TERMS

British cooking term	American equivalent	British cooking term	American equivalent
aubergine	eggplant	jam	jelly
bacon rasher	Canadian bacon	jug	pitcher
baking beans	pie weights	kitchen paper	paper towel
baking parchment	parchment paper	minced meat	ground meat
beetroot	beet	mixed spice	allspice
bicarbonate of soda	baking soda	mould	mold
black pudding	blood sausage	nozzle	decorating tip
cake tin	cake pan	ovenproof	heatproof
chilli	chili	paper cases	paper baking cups
chocolate, plain dark	bittersweet chocolate	pastry case	pie crust
choux pastry	cream puff paste	piping bag	pastry bag
cider	hard cider	polenta	stone-ground cornmeal
cling film	plastic wrap	red pepper	red bell pepper
coriander	cilantro	rocket	arugula
cornflour	cornstarch	spring onion	green onion/scallion
cornmeal	cornflour	stone	pit
cream, double	heavy cream	sugar, icing	confectioners' sugar
cream, single	light cream	sugar, caster	superfine sugar
desiccated coconut	shredded, dried coconut	sugar, demerara	turbinado sugar
digestive biscuits	graham crackers	sugar, dark muscovado	dark brown sugar
essence	extract	sugar, light muscovado	light brown sugar
fillet steak	filet mignon	sultanas	golden raisins
flaked almonds	slivered almonds	swede	rutabaga
flour, plain	all-purpose flour	sweetcorn	corn
flour, self-raising	self-rising flour	Swiss roll tin	jelly roll pan
flour, strong	bread flour	unfiltered apple juice	apple cider
frying pan	skillet	vanilla pod	vanilla bean
gammon	ham	whisk	beat
golden syrup	light corn syrup	wire rack	cooling rack
grill	broiler	yeast, fast-action dried	active dry yeast
heaped tablespoon	heaping tablespoon		

AN ABUNDANCE OF THANKS

There are so many people I wish to thank, not only for their help with this book but for the constant support through a varied and sometimes incredibly challenging career! So listen up:

Special thanks to David Lynch: For creating this wonderful and strange world that continues to inspire and astound. I thank you so dearly.

And Mark Frost: Again for creating this magical world of *Twin Peaks* and inspiring so many, thank you.

Sallie Ankers, my big big sister: For always having a level head and a dry sense of humour and for always helping me see all sides and finding good Christmas fairs!

Angela Bowden, my big sister: For always making me laugh until the point of crying and being able to see the humour in an unhumourous situation!

Rod Bowden, my bro: For always being true to who you are and what you have achieved. Your strength is incredible and your talent is admirable.

Mark Ankers, the best brother-in-law anyone could ever have: For always telling me that as long as I'm happy, that's all that matters.

Emma Ankers: For growing into a beautiful young woman who I'm so proud to call my niece. For your care and warmth and loyalty.

Georgia Ankers: For being strong and always supportive of my work. Also for being perfect company for cream tea when I'm craving it! I'm proud to have a niece like you.

Kurtis Bowden: For being able to have a smirk in any situation. You're a wonderful nephew and I'm so proud of what you have achieved this past couple of years.

Jack Bowden: For bringing the rock and being awesome! Never cut your hair!

Adrian Bowden & Jacqui Canham: For your constant support, wonderful friendship and provision of my funniest cat/mouse story to date! You are truly two of the finest people in my life.

Sarah Close: For being the main lady, allowing me to be my crazy self, never judging me for ridiculous decisions I've made and always being there at the end of the phone. When's your birthday again?

Sarah Styles: For kicking my butt when I've needed it and talking sense when I've been buzzing like a crazy woman. You are one of the strongest women I know and my life is richer for you.

Lynda Bowley (née Gale): For taking a 17 year old and giving her confidence and the best friend someone could ever have. Also for being the only person I've drunk a bottle of Southern Comfort for breakfast with – I miss those days!

Clare Evers: For being as crazy as I am and understanding the crazy! Genuinely one of the most wonderful people put on this earth and I'm thankful you are in my life.

Bernie Byrnes: For being the first person to give me confidence to go for what I want and what I'm passionate about, and for allowing me to start to grow into who I was to become.

Marina Caldarone: For being the next Bernie! For seeing through my tough times and seeing the person underneath and bringing that to the surface. Your friendship knows no bounds and I am so grateful for you being in my life. Also for all the weird food you make me!

John Dryden: For seeing something in me so long ago that you developed and supported. And giving me the year that is still the best of my life with the best people.

Sally Wood: My sister from another mister! You are divine, and a true friend and so dear to my heart. Your front room was the cosiest place I ever lived and time and time again you have supported, advised and laughed with me. There's seriously no one better to eat a ton of cakes with!

Ronnie Wood: For making my beautiful friend so happy and supplying me with copious amounts of great coffee!

John Cole: For being my brother from another mother and always having faith in me – and for one of the funniest motorway drives I've ever had to this day.

Daniel Fearn: For being the only person I genuinely feel happy jumping around to *House of Pain* with!

Karen Petersen: For being a wonderful friend and partner in crime and providing me with some of the funniest moments of my life…bottled face not included (slightly included)!

Martin Craig: For being my wonderful friend, your incredible loyalty and believing in me.

Guy Thompson: Hocus Pocus Focus, there's nothing more to say.

Andrew Walker: Simply for being you…and the perfect Take That to my Lulu.

Laura Hawley: For being a wonderful friend whose love is unconditional.

Robin Walton: For being there at the very beginning with tremendous support and friendship.

Shira Macleod: For allowing me to experiment and supporting me in my crazy ideas…that somehow worked! And for providing insight when I've needed it.

Duncan Stewart: For being a great support to me and the fest, and always having a door open for a chat… or a cuddle (with Rufus).

Bobbi Blackman: For allowing me to sleep on dressing room sofas when I was exhausted from working five jobs! And for the wonderful chats over tea and chocolates!

Rosie Greatorex: For being one of the most beautiful souls I know, and for your support.

Nik Whybrew: For all your support and advice when I've needed it – no one wears a cardigan like you.

Stacey Smith: For your support in the early days, for seeing the potential and going the extra mile.

Calvin Brown: For your never-ending loyalty.

Kathryn Davies: For your wonderful friendship, ear and support.

Craig Prentice: For your support and for giving us the best view in London year after year!

Charlotte Goodman: For your support and for providing good entertainment for our guests!

Amanda Hicks & Jared Lyon: For your brilliant support when I started out and your wonderful advice and encouragement. Amanda – also for your hair, that stuff is outrageous!

Josh Eisenstadt: For your support, your friendship and your incredible mind!

Rob & Deanne Lindley: For continuing the great support after Amanda & Jared handed over to you. You're great pals and I'm happy we have the trust in each other that we do.

Gina Lee Ronhovde: For your support…and the candy package!

Michael Barile: For your amazing support and belief in me and the fest!

Madchen Amick: For being a truly wonderful supporter and beautiful friend with an inspiring soul. Your belief and support of me is unparalleled and I love you dearly.

Sheryl Lee: For having an open heart and believing in me and what I do. I truly believe you are one of the kindest souls I have had the pleasure to know.

Al Strobel: For making me smile and for your support. Our chats are one of my favourite things and I adore the way you cherish this world.

Sherilyn Fenn: For your support, your positivity and for making me roar with laughter after just five minutes of your brilliant company!

Lenny Von Dohlen: For your support and your good heart and friendship.

Catherine E. Coulson: For being there at a time when I was at my most fragile and for your wonderful support. You are so missed.

Charlotte Stewart: For your wonderful support. Nothing is ever too much for you and I love your warmth and friendship.

Dana Ashbrook: For your huge support and for giving so much to the fans and me, and your never-ending positivity!

Ian Buchanan: For your friendship and support. The next Starbucks is on me.

James Marshall: For your support. I can't wait to have you here!

Phoebe Augustine & Stephen Ceresia: For your support and wonderful company in London. Cannot wait to hang with you guys again.

Julee Cruise: For your support and your commitment to your fans.

Kimmy Robertson: For your beautiful soul, your support and, of course, your brilliant friendship and innovative tacos!

Jen Lynch: For your support and inspiration for our Legend of Lynch day – you were with us in spirit in 2015!

Mina Tobias: For joining us in London and being so wonderful to have at the fest, gracing us with your music and soulful spirit.

The rest of the amazing cast of *Twin Peaks*: For your inspiration, your wonderful characters and making this world so real for so many.

Holly McGee at Java Distribution: For your support and enthusiasm…and our coffee quest!

Gabby & Veronica at CBS: For your support, guidance and encouragement and seeing the potential in us. Here's to a very exciting future!

NBC Universal, especially Louise Watson: For your incredible support and for always having the most wonderful smile on your face!

Steve White: For being there from the very beginning and seeing the potential, and for your constant support ever since!

5th Column Printing: For your constant support; we're proud to partner with you each year.

Riverside Studios, especially Guy Hornsby & William Burdett-Coutts: For allowing me to develop the *Twin Peaks* UK Festival and still supporting it even when we moved venues. You will always be our first wonderful home.

Tyrone Walker-Hebborn & Genesis Cinema: For your warm welcome, providing us with an outstanding venue and allowing us to transform it into a *Twin Peaks*-inspired setting. You have a fantastic team who revelled in everything *Twin Peaks* with us, and you hold a special place in our hearts.

Picturehouse Central, Chloe, Toby, Claire, Darren and Micallar: For believing and trusting in us and allowing us to be part of your beautiful new venue. But not for the cakes in the café, as they will be the death of me!

My amazing team (from all the years!)

Rose Thorne & Benjamin Louche: There are not enough thank yous for everything you have contributed and for the wonderful friendship you have given me. I'm so proud of what we have created together and I'm excited about what we will achieve in the future.

Tom Huddleston: There is so much to thank you for, you wonderful, wonderful person. I'm so pleased we have taken this journey together since the beginning. Or is this only the beginning? Thank you.

Mark Swan: For being my rock, being you…and believing in me.

Helen Henson: For being there at the very beginnings and helping me grow. You're a wonderful friend and rockin' mother!

Sophie Ralli: For your hard work and dedication, your humour, your wonderful insight and friendship. I couldn't have done 2015 without you.

Kitty Edgar: For your huge dedication and your brilliant friendship, and the ability to have the best hilarious outlook in any situation!

Claire Laffar: Your commitment and artistry have been a vital part of the fest, as have your wonderful knowledge and friendship, thank you.

Marc Brown: No words my friend – you're a superstar and a major cog in the machinery!

Steve Richley: Utterly brilliant to have the chance to work with you again! Thank you for all your work on the fest, here's to the future bud!

Kerry Rush: You've been with me since the beginning and nothing is ever too much trouble for you. What you have achieved over the last few years is wondrous and you will only get stronger from here.

Quinn Patrick: For your wonderful friendship, your unparalleled loyalty and your positive light. You are one of the dearest people to me in this crazy world and I value our friendship more than you could know.

Kevin Millington: From Riverside to *Twin Peaks*, your loyalty is unparalleled and I'm thankful for your friendship and support.

Cam Mitchell: You took us from Riverside and created a beautiful setting at our new venue, facing trying challenges but delivering in every way, thank you.

Sandy Gunn: We'll always have 2010…I believe our friendship was solidified forever!

Roger Galpin: For being our hero!

Derek MacKenzie: For being our other hero!

Steven Reed: For looking after all our fabulous customers for the first few fests. I admire your strength and positivity through very trying times – you are a star Panda!

Gareth Gatrell: For your stunning photography and even more stunning friendship.

Stuart Meredith: For your wonderful designs, your support and for being there when I needed you.

Simon Ellis: For your support and sterling work.

Will Scothard: For your stunning film work in 2010 and 2011.

Christian Herrman: For producing a fabulous film for us in 2012.

Nicolai Kornum: For your brilliant work on our 2013 and 2014 films.

Anthony Ratcliffe: For your constant support throughout the years and creating a great film for us in 2015.

James Arden: For your slick work on our other 2015 film and your constant professionalism.

Michael Eppy: For believing in us and being a fantastic support.

Everyone at Octopus Books, especially Eleanor Maxfield and Yasia Williams-Leedham: For giving me the opportunity to bring this book to the *Twin Peaks* fans and for your guidance and belief in what we could achieve. You are incredible women with brilliant vision, thank you!

Annie Nichols: For your wonderful work on this book, I'm super-excited about taking this journey with you! And donuts, I'm super-excited about those too!

Addie Chin: For turning our recipes into stunningly perfect photos. Working with you on the shoot was a blast. Your eye and love of *Twin Peaks* produced the most wonderful results. Thank you so much for bringing your best to the table!

And to all the *Twin Peaks* fans: You are what makes this world of *Twin Peaks* so special and I thank you for all the support you have shown and your excitement about this book. I hope you enjoy it!

And Chester: For distracting me constantly from work!

And for my darling Ciaran & Jonathan Masters (née O'keeffe AKA Colin), Jack & Molly: I have no words but thank you, I love you.

PICTURE CREDITS

Lindsey Bowden 6 above right. **Dreamstime.com** Alexander Pladdet 123 above right; Eskymaks 140; Picsfive 123 below left; Saknakorn 61; stockcreations 81; Svetlana Day 123 below right. **Joseph Tovey Frost** 211 above right. **Gareth Gatrell** 6 above right, below right, 210 below right, 211 above left, 211 below left. **Nicolai Kornum** 210 left, 211 below right. **Shutterstock** Fotokor77 19. **Soulstealer** 212, 213. **StockFood** Colin Cooke 123 above left. **Amy T. Zielinski** 6 above left, centre left, below left.

Fashion photography pages 20–25 supplied by Dreamstime.com and iStockphoto.com.

PROPS

The Publisher would like to thank the following for kindly loaning us props for the photography:

Mojo Margate
www.mojomargate.com

Fontaine Decorative
www.fontainedecorative.com

Duke St Diner
https://www.facebook.com/dinermargate/

Lindsey Bowden was born in Portsmouth in 1976, the youngest of four children. She moved to London in 1996 and worked as an actress after graduating from drama school. However, she soon found herself drawn more to creating work, so pursued a career in producing.

For a number of years, Lindsey combined her producing with running top UK music/theatre venues in London and Edinburgh, including the legendary Roundhouse in Camden and the historic Riverside Studios in Hammersmith. It was while working at Riverside Studios that Lindsey founded the *Twin Peaks* UK Festival. She has also worked with exciting companies such as Circomlombia, The Jim Henson Company and the Royal Shakespeare Company on their celebrated Histories season.

A self-confessed workaholic, Lindsey's favourite place to unwind is anywhere by the sea and she can often be found sitting on a beach in the middle of winter. She also loves watching *Scooby Doo* cartoons, and of course indulging in her favourite episodes of *Twin Peaks*.

INDEX

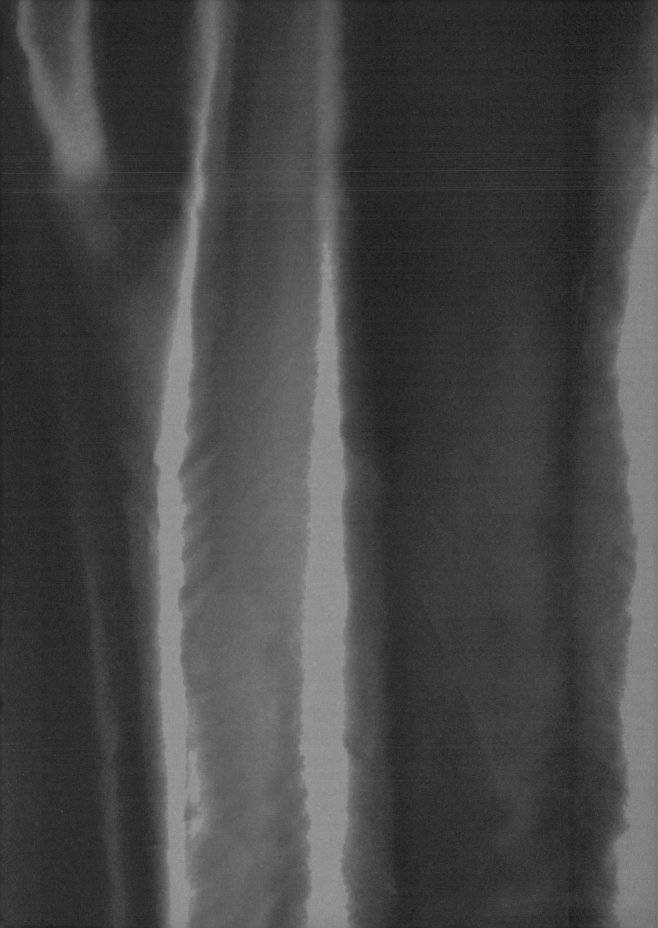